Pharmacy Management Software

for Pharmacy Technicians

A WORKTEXT

Pharmacy Management Software

for Pharmacy Technicians

A WORKTEXT

DAA Enterprises, Inc.
Brookline, Massachusetts

Written By
Karen Davis, BHS, CPhT
Accreditation Consultant
Society for the Education of Pharmacy Technicians (SEPhT) Founder

THIRD EDITION

ELSEVIER

ELSEVIER

3251 Riverport Lane
St. Louis, Missouri 63043

PHARMACY MANAGEMENT SOFTWARE FOR PHARMACY TECHNICIANS,   ISBN: 978-0-323-42832-3
THIRD EDITION

Notices

International Standard Book Number: 978-0-323-42832-3

Director, Private Sector Education: Jennifer Janson
Senior Content Strategist: Kristin Wilhelm
Content Development Manager: Luke Held
Content Development Specialist: Kelly Skelton
Publishing Services Manager: Jeff Patterson
Design Direction: Julia Dummitt

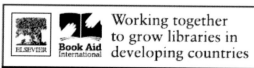

Printed in Canada
Last digit is the print number: 9 8 7 6 5 4 3 2 1

Preface

Welcome to the exciting world of pharmacy technology! You have started on a journey into one of today's fastest growing fields in health care. Whether you end up working in an institutional pharmacy, a community pharmacy, one of the large pharmacy chain stores, or in another specialty field, the skills that you will gain from *Pharmacy Management Software for Pharmacy Technicians* will help prepare you for your new career.

New federal regulations now require pharmacists to spend more time with patients providing patient education; as a result, pharmacy technicians are increasingly asked to perform duties traditionally fulfilled by pharmacists. Because of the nature of the pharmacy technician's work, hands-on training is critically important in educational programs. This software package is designed to provide hands-on training and help you master the information and skills necessary to be a successful pharmacy technician. The various activities will challenge your knowledge, help further reinforce key concepts, and allow you to gauge your understanding of the subject matter studied in your pharmacy technician program.

With the continued expansion of the pharmacy technician role and the potential for specialty roles, the need for advanced education is increasing. Simulated practice to prepare a competitive workforce requires a reliable and understandable resource, which is correlated with the goals of the American Society of Health-System Pharmacists (ASHP) and the Pharmacy Technician Certification Exam (PTCE) domains. *Pharmacy Management Software for Pharmacy Technicians* has been correlated to ASHP goals and objectives and is specifically written for the pharmacy technician student. New labs, such as automated cabinet dispensing, prescription verification using bar code scanning, as well as patient profiles and medication therapy management, adjudication and inventory, and nonsterile compounding, are now included.

The worktext is divided into four sections: Community Pharmacy Practice, Institutional Pharmacy Practice, Additional Practice Settings, and Documentation. Each section guides you through the various tasks that pharmacy technicians are expected to perform in that setting—first in isolation and then in sequential hands-on activities performed in a simulated lab.

Contents

SECTION II: INSTITUTIONAL PHARMACY PRACTICE

SECTION III: ADDITIONAL PRACTICE SETTINGS

SECTION IV: DOCUMENTATION

Installing and Navigating Visual SuperScript

INSTALLATION

The software, along with installation instructions, is available on the Evolve Resources site at http://evolve.elsevier.com/pharmmanagement/PT/.

THE BASICS

Understanding the basics of software navigation is essential to your success in this course. If you are already familiar with Microsoft Windows applications, such as Word or Excel, then you already have the necessary basic navigation knowledge. However, even if you are new to using a computer, you should be able to navigate the software after learning a few key concepts.

The Visual SuperScript manual is designed to teach the functions of the software in different Lab exercises. Each section covers a specific practice area and the tasks performed in that area. With the data entry instructions, the hands-on or simulation laboratory experience is then incorporated to teach the tasks that you will need to practice.

Similar to baking, you should follow the Lab in a step-by-step direction, just as you would a recipe. The directions are a guide through the functions of the screens and tabs within the software.

The Lab exercises also allow for practice in areas required by the American Society of Health-System Pharmacists (ASHP) training programs. Typed and handwritten prescriptions and orders are provided for interpretation. In addition, simulated comprehensive exercises for community and institutional settings have been included for scenarios and team laboratory practice sessions with several handwritten prescriptions and institutional orders. These prescriptions and orders will enable you to simulate laboratory exercises before on-the-job training, using real-life scenarios and *real* prescriptions used in the community and institutional settings.

GETTING STARTED

The first screen that you will see after installing the software is the main menu. When you click on a menu choice that appears across the top of the main menu, you will see a drop-down list. Each menu choice on that drop-down list appears with one letter underlined. That letter represents a *hot key* for that choice. Each item on the menu may be selected by pressing the *Alt key* and the corresponding hot key at the same time. For example, an *Activity Summary* may be selected from the **REPORTS/ ADMIN REPORTS** menu by pressing on the A key. Of course, you may also select any menu option by moving the mouse pointer to it and clicking on it.

Note: Unless indicated otherwise, *clicking the mouse* or *clicking on it* means clicking the left mouse button once. On certain occasions, you will need to click the left button twice quickly, which is called *double clicking*. Certain features of the program are accessed through menus that are displayed by clicking the right mouse button once, which is called *right clicking*.

Objects, Icons, and Controls

You will interact with the software by using the various objects that appear in each dialog box. Some objects appear as buttons with small pictures on them. These will be referred to as *icons*. Other objects appear as *check boxes* or *drop-down lists*, and simple data entry areas are referred to as *data entry fields* or *text boxes*.

In most dialog boxes, data can be entered in multiple ways. Several text boxes and a few check boxes may be offered. The blinking cursor will provide a visual clue as to where you are in the form. To move from one space on a form to another, pressing the TAB key is best.

Data Entry Fields

Data entry fields are the most common objects that you will encounter. They are used to type in data or to display numbers, such as names, Drug Enforcement Administration (DEA) numbers, and dates. Examples of data entry fields are the *Rx No.*, *Disp Date*, and *RPH Initials* boxes on the *Prescription Processing form*.

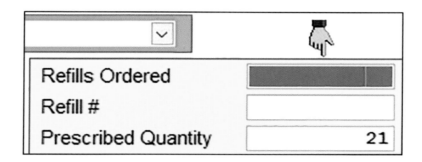

Some data entry fields may be *read-only*, which means they can only display information. In read-only data entry fields, information cannot be added or changed.

Buttons

Buttons are function keys that open dialog boxes when clicked.

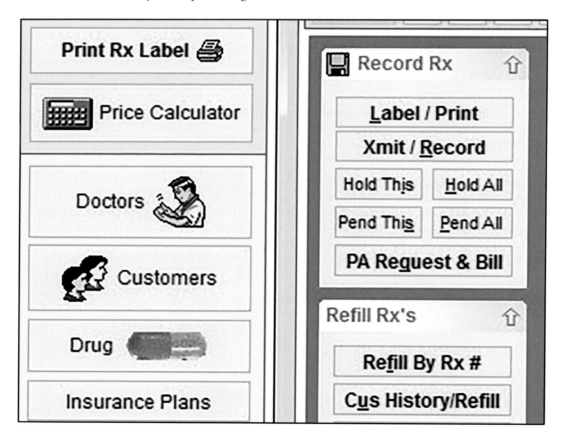

Drop-Down Lists

Drop-down lists are used only when certain responses can be used for a specific part of a form. Each drop-down list has a downward small arrow next to it. You can see what choices you have for a data entry field by clicking on the downward arrow and then clicking on the response of your choice. For example, when entering the origin of the prescription, the user clicks on the arrow to the right of the *Rx Origin* data entry field and then selects from the choices in the drop-down list.

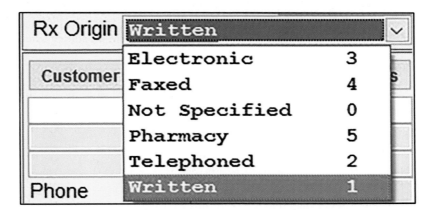

Some drop-down lists have content that can be changed, added, or removed. Each drop-down list has a downward arrow with line below it, instead of only the arrow by itself.

Icons

Icons, or buttons with pictures on them, appear throughout the software. However, you will mostly see icons on the **FILE NAVIGATION TOOLBAR** that appears at the top of your screen.

All of these buttons appear whenever a form is being used that is designed for data entry. These buttons are referred to as the *navigation tools*, and the bar on which they appear is called the *toolbar*.

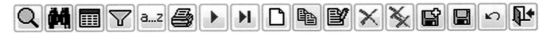

Each button has a picture that provides a clue about its function. A slightly more detailed explanation of the button's purpose may be obtained by moving the mouse pointer to a button and then holding it there for several seconds. A small description of the button will appear.
The toolbar icons and corresponding purposes are as follows:

FIND button: Is used to help find records.

LOCATE button: Is used to locate records that meet certain criteria, such as families that live in a certain Zip code.

LIST button: Enables you to display the records in a file as a list.

FILTER button: Allows you to set filters so that only certain subsets of records are displayed. The filter function is similar to the locate function.

SORT button: Allows you to select the order in which records are displayed.

PRINT button: Allows you to print the record(s) that you are currently viewing.

NEXT button: Moves you to the next record in a table.

LAST button: Moves you to the last record in a table.

NEW button: Displays a blank form to begin adding a new record.

Copy button: Makes a copy of the current record and displays it for editing. This feature is handy when most of the information on a newly created record can be carried over from another record.

Edit button: Allows you to make changes to a record.

Delete button: Deletes the current record.

Group Delete button: Allows a group of records that meet a certain criterion to be deleted.

More button: Saves the current record and displays a blank form for adding a new record.

Save button: Saves the current record.

Cancel button: Cancels all changes made to the current record since the last time the record was saved.

Close button: Closes the form.

TIPS

- Using your **Tab** key is better than the mouse for this software. Most prescription software is **Tab** driven.
- When you are trying to enter information into a field, make sure it is **BLUE** or **RED**, which signals that the field is ready for entry of data.
- Always enter the first three letters when **SEARCHING**. Entering too much information will limit the choices made available in the resulting window.
- Use the **Logout** button to exit the program, rather than the **File** and **Exit** buttons at the top.

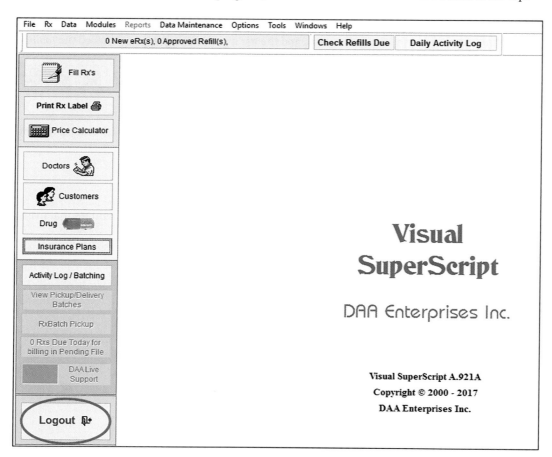

- Because you want to be efficient and save time when performing data entry, use abbreviations as much as possible, which will prepare you for on-the-job experiences.
- When saving a prescription, two choices are provided at the top left.
    1. The **SAVE** 🖫 option will keep the prescription you just filled and allows you to start from a fresh screen or patient.
    2. If you have more than one prescription for the same patient, the **MORE** 🖫 option will keep some prefilled information in the screen for you. This option is designed to save time in the data entry process.

Reinforcing Skills (American Society of Health-System Pharmacists Sequential Learning)

The Visual SuperScript manual is designed to teach the functions of automated simulation software by using detailed specific or isolated Lab exercises. Once the individual data entry functions are taught, including managing electronic profiles and medication review, inventory and third-party reporting, narcotics, compounding, and distribution, the hands-on skill of processing or preparing the medication is performed in each Lab exercise. The newly designed laboratory manual and software are designed to incorporate computer skills with the tasks performed in both community and institutional practices, by adding data entry with simulation using actual equipment and supplies found in the pharmacy practice.

Once each task that pharmacy technicians are required to practice in an American Society of Health-System Pharmacists (ASHP)–based program are separately demonstrated, the manual provides the opportunity to combine the comprehensive functions learned in the software program with tasks performed in those areas, **sequentially**. Instructors can use role play, teams, or interdisciplinary means to require the student to practice all required tasks in a controlled environment, from start to finish, as in a real-world scenario, before participating in their externship experience.

Using the database throughout the entire program in a simulated laboratory pharmacy and in conjunction with the proper equipment and supplies allows the trainee to complete and retain the documentation of skills needed before entering the pharmacy workforce.

Excerpt from ASHP standards:

While each skill is taught in isolation, by the end of the simulated component, students must perform each skill in a sequential manner the way it is performed in a pharmacy...

Sig Abbreviation Shortcuts

ABBREVIATION	MEANING	ABBREVIATION	MEANING
1-2	1 or 2	$D_{10}W$	Dextrose 10% in water
1-2G	1 or 2 drops	$D_{20}W$	Dextrose 20% in water
1APP	1 applicator	$D_{30}W$	Dextrose 30% in water
1C	1 capsule	$D_{40}W$	Dextrose 40% in water
1CBID	Take 1 capsule twice each day	$D_{50}W$	Dextrose 50% in water
1CQD	Take 1 capsule daily	$D_{70}W$	Dextrose 70% in water
1CQID	Take 1 capsule four times a day	D	Daily
1CTID	Take 1 capsule three times a day	D1T	Dissolve 1 tablet
1DR	Take 1 teaspoon	DA	Dissolve and
1G	1 drop	DAY	Day
1IAPP	Insert 1 applicator	DIA	Diarrhea
1SSTS	Take 1½ teaspoons	DIS	Dissolve
1T	1 tablet	DISP	Dispense
1TBID	1 tablet twice a day	DR	Drink
1TPOBID	1 tablet by mouth twice a day	DX	Diagnosis
1TPOQD	1 tablet by mouth each day	DWW	Dilute with water
1TPOQDHS	1 tablet by mouth every day at bedtime	EN	Each nostril
1TQD	1 tablet each day	EVERY	Every
1TQID	1 tablet four times a day	F	For
1TTID	1 tablet three times a day	F1	For 1 week
2C	2 capsules	F10	For 10 days
2G	2 drops	F14	For 14 days
2T	2 tablets	F2	For 2 weeks
3G	3 drops	F5	For 5 days
3TSP	3 teaspoons	F7	For 7 days
4G	4 drops	FE	For external use only
4HRS	4 hours	FIN	Finished
AA	Affected area; Amino acid solution	FP	For pain
AAA	Apply to affected area	FX	Fracture
AAD	After dinner	GTT	Drop
AAS	After supper	GTTS	Drops
AC	Before meals	(H)	Hypodermic
AE	Into the affected eye	H, HR	Hour
AM	Morning	HA	Headache
AND	And	HOUR	Hour
AP	Apply	I	Instill
ASAP	As soon as possible	I1G	Instill 1 drop
ATC	Around the clock	I1P	Inhale 1 puff
BID	Twice a day	I1S	Insert 1 suppository
BM	Bowel movement	I1T	Insert 1 tablet
BOLUS	Intravenous push	I2G	Instill 2 drops
BP	Blood pressure	I2P	Inhale 2 puffs
BRP	Bathroom priv.	I3G	Instill 3 drops
C	With	I3P	Inhale 3 puffs
CAP	Capsule	I4G	Instill 4 drops
CCM	With food or milk	I4P	Inhale 4 puffs
CF	With food	I5G	Instill 5 drops
CM	With meals	ID	Intradermal
D_5W	Dextrose 5% in water	IM	Intramuscular
D_5 ¼ N.S.	Dextrose 5% in ¼ normal saline	INFECT	Infection
D_5 0.2% NACL	Dextrose 5% in 0.2% sodium chloride	IL	In liquids
D_5 ½ N.S.	Dextrose 5% in ½ normal saline	INF	For infection
D_5 0.45% NACL	Dextrose 5% in 0.45% sodium chloride	INS	Insert
D_5 N.S.	Dextrose 5% in normal saline	IT	Intrathecal
D_5 0.9%	Dextrose 5% in 0.9% sodium chloride	ITCH	Itching
D_5LR	Dextrose 5% in lactated Ringer's solution	IV	Intravenous
		IVP	Intravenous push
		IVPB	IV piggyback

Continued.

Sig Abbreviation Shortcuts—cont'd

ABBREVIATION	MEANING	ABBREVIATION	MEANING
IVSS	IV soluset	SSTSP	½ teaspoon
IW	In water	STAT	Immediately
L	Left	SUB-Q	Subcutaneously
LE	Left ear	SX	Surgery
LR (RL)	Lactated Ringer's solution (Ringer's lactated solution)	T	Take
		T1	Take 1
MR	May repeat	T1C	Take 1 capsule
N	Nerves	T1-2C	Take 1 or 2 capsules
NF	Nonformulary	T1-2T	Take 1 or 2 tablets
NKA	No known allergies	T1SST	Take 1½ tablets
NPO	Nothing by mouth	TID	Three times a day
NR	No refill	T1TBL	Take 1 tablespoonful
N.S.	Normal saline	T1TSP	Take 1 teaspoonful
NV	Nausea and vomiting	T2	Take 2
(O)	Orally	T2C	Take 2 capsules
OA	Into affected eye	T2TSP	Take 2 teaspoons
P	For pain, after	T2T	Take 2 tablets
PIT	Place 1 tablet	T3	Take 3
PA	Pain	T3C	Take 3 capsules
PAC	Packet	T3T	Take 3 tablets
PATCH	Patch	T3TSP	Take 3 teaspoons
PC	After meals	T4C	Take 4 capsules
PL	Place	T4T	Take 4 tablets
PM	Afternoon	T4TSP	Take 4 teaspoons
PO	By mouth	T5C	Take 5 capsules
PR	Rectally	T5T	Take 5 tablets
PRN	As needed	TAKE	Take
PRNA	As needed for anxiety	TBID	Take 1 tablet twice a day
PRNC	As needed for cough	TBL	Tablespoonful
PRND	As needed for diarrhea	TBSP	Tablespoonful
PRNF	As needed for	THEN	Then
PRNHA	As needed for headache	TID	Three times a day
PRNP	As needed for pain	TK	Take
PV	Vaginally	TLA	To large area
Q	Every	TOP	Topically
Q12H	Every 12 hours	TPN	Total parenteral nutrition
Q3-4H	Every 3 to 4 hours	TRA	To run at
Q4-6H	Every 4 to 6 hours	TSP	Teaspoonful
Q4H	Every 4 hours	TSST	Take ½ tablet
Q6-8H	Every 6 to 8 hours	TUD	Take as directed
Q6H	Every 6 hours	TTSP	Take ½ teaspoonful
Q8H	Every 8 hours	U2I	Use 2 inhalations
QAM	Every morning	U2P	Use 2 puffs
QH	Every hour	U2S	Use 2 sprays
QID	Four times a day	UAT	Until all taken
QNOC	Every night	UD	As directed, unit dose
QOH	Every other hour	UF	Until finished
QPM	Every evening	UG	Until gone
QS	Sufficient quantity	USE	Use
QSAD	Sufficient quantity to add	USP	United States Pharmacopeia
R	Right	UUD	Use as directed
RE	Right ear	VAG	Vaginally
RX	Take, recipe	W/A	While awake
S	Suppository, without	WF	With food
S2D	Squirt twice daily	WJ	With juice
SIG	Label	WM	With meal
SL	Under tongue	WM	With meals and bedtime
SSAP	½ applicator	WW	With water

Section I

Community Pharmacy Practice

INTRODUCTION TO THE WORKFLOW OF COMMUNITY PHARMACY PRACTICE

Community pharmacy practice includes pharmacies that dispense medications to customers who are usually ambulatory and able to take their own medications. The technician's role consists of working directly with customers and other health care professionals, insurance processing and data entry, inventory control, pharmacology, laws and regulations, and record keeping. The practice may be in a retail, franchise, or independent pharmacy, and all work is performed under the direct supervision of a pharmacist. Each state has specific rules and regulations, but the technician works directly with the customers and pharmacists every day.

The Lab exercises in this section provide detailed steps to teach the technician how to use the Visual SuperScript software applications for entering prescriptions and maintaining and editing patient information in the electronic profile, including all aspects of prescription processing from interpretation to a finished product.

The workflow for a community practice starts with the customer. By simulating each function in isolation and then combining the sequences, as teams or with partners, Visual SuperScript provides real-world practice in the lab setting before entering the externship phase of your training.

Nonsterile or *extemporaneous compounding* and dispensing of over-the-counter (OTC) medications and durable and nondurable supplies and equipment are also common tasks that the technician performs in a retail setting; these tasks are also included in this section. Labs include the label and data entry processes for common compound types and include hands-on exercises to create each form using simulated medications.

LAB 1

Adding a Physician or Prescriber to the Database

■ Introduction

When working in a community practice setting, typically you will service patients who will be prescribed medications for either a 30- or a 90-day supply. Pain or antibiotic medications for a shorter number of days or amounts may also be prescribed for patients.

Physicians can telephone, fax, or e-prescribe (electronically submit) a prescription to your pharmacy, or send a patient to hand carry a prescription to the counter. These prescribers can be from community clinics, physician's offices, hospitals, and even out of town or state. A checksum test determines whether a Drug Enforcement Administration (DEA) number is false or valid. Physician prescribers will have a nine-character code, and the beginning two characters will be an A, B, F, M, or X. In addition, other disciplines, such as nurse practitioners, veterinarians, and psychologists can also write prescriptions. As an example, for a nurse practitioner, an "M" may be assigned as part of his or her DEA number. The number, which can be mathematically verified, must be on the prescription if a controlled substance is prescribed.

Example: Dr. Jack Jenkins (AJ3456781)

FIRST: *Verify that the initials are correct. The first letter should be one of the DEA-approved designations used for a physician, and in this case an A is present. The second letter should be the first initial of the last name, which in this case is J.*

Step 1: *Add the first, third, and fifth digits: 3 + 5 + 7 = 15*
Step 2: *Add the second, fourth, and sixth digits: 4 + 6 + 8 = 18*
Step 3: *Multiply the number obtained in Step 2 times 2: 18 × 2 = 36*
Step 4: *Add the numbers obtained in Steps 1 and 3: 15 + 36 = 51*

If this DEA number is valid, then the last digit of the DEA number should be 1, and it is.

MEDICATION SAFETY CONSIDERATION

Always be aware of the signature and DEA number on a prescription, especially on a prescription for a controlled substance. If the checksum method does not work, then the pharmacist (not the patient) should be immediately notified.

■ Lab Objectives

In this Lab, you will:

- Perform the checksum method to verify the DEA number for a prescriber.
- Demonstrate the steps required to add a physician or prescriber to the database, using software data entry skills in a simulated laboratory environment.
- Verify each other's work (simulate the tech-check-tech [TCT]) when verifying a physician DEA number and prescriber entry information.

ASHP goals: 3, 8, 12, 17, 18, 35, 36, and 41.

■ Scenario

Today, you are working in a simulated retail setting and learning to add new physicians to the database.

The Lab exercise will teach you how to perform the steps of entering a new prescriber, and you will then be given several additional prescribers to enter in the exercise. Check each prescriber for the validity of the DEA number using the example (steps) provided in the Introduction of this Lab, and note any DEA numbers that are not valid. Ask another student to check your math; if you still believe a number is not valid, then alert your instructor.

Enter all the information listed for each new physician to ensure that future prescriptions you enter will have complete information for each prescriber.

■ Student Directions

Estimated completion time: 30 minutes

1. Read through the steps in the Lab before performing the Lab exercise.
2. After reading through the Lab, perform the required steps to enter provider information.
3. Complete the exercise at the end of the Lab.

Dr. Larry Peterson
11321 9th Street
Guthrie Center, IA 50115
Office: (717) 330-1990, ext. 109
Fax: (717) 330-1991

Date: _____

Patient Name: _____

Address: _____

Rx

Refill: _____

Product Selection Permitted   Dispense As Written

DEA: BP1234892
State License: 073223   _____
                                                                   M.D.

STEPS TO ADD A PHYSICIAN OR PRESCRIBER TO THE DATABASE

1. Access the main screen of Visual SuperScript.

2. Click on the **DOCTORS** button located on the left side of the screen. A dialog box entitled *Doctors* will pop up.

3. Click on the **FIND** 🔍 icon located on the top left of the toolbar. A dialog box entitled *Doctor Lookup* will pop up.

4. Enter the first three letters of the prescriber's last name in the **NAME** field.

5. If the physician is not found in the list, then click **ADD**. The form is now ready for you to enter the prescriber information.

 LAB TIP

You may type the first three letters of the physician's last name and press **ENTER**. If the prescriber is not in the database, then click **ADD** at the bottom of the dialog box. You will be asked whether you want to add the doctor manually. Click **YES** to add the new prescriber.

6. The **NAME** is a required field. Enter the prescriber name starting with the last name, followed by a comma, one space, and then the first name.

Enter *Peterson, Larry* for Dr. Larry Peterson.

 LAB TIP

Enter all names EXACTLY as described above. First name followed by a comma, one space, then the last name. To search for a particular name or drug, **always enter only the FIRST three letters**, which saves time in a busy pharmacy. If the name or drug is completely typed, then you run the risk of misspelling the item, which will not allow you to find a particular name or drug.

7. The **CONTACT** field should contain the name of the person you usually speak with when you call the physician's office for refill authorization. Enter *Brandon* as the contact.

8. Enter the prescriber's **ADDRESS**.

Enter *11321 9th Street, Guthrie Center, IA 50115* as the address.

9. Click the arrow to the right of the Zip code field to ensure that your Zip code is in the database. The *Zip* dialog box will open. If your Zip code is there, click **OK** and advance to Step 11.

   Note: If the Zip code is in the database, then the city and state fields will automatically populate.

10. If the Zip code you typed is not found, you will need to add the city and the Zip code to the database. Within the *Zip* dialog box, click **ADD**.

   a. A pop-up dialog box appears entitled *Zip Codes*.

   b. Enter the prescriber Zip code, city, and state postal abbreviation.

11. Enter the prescriber's **PHONE** information.

Enter *717/330-1990 extension 109* as the office phone.
Enter *717/330-1991* as the fax number.

12. Enter the prescriber's initials in the **QUICK CODE** field.

13. Enter *BP1234892* as the **DEA** number.

14. Verify the **DEA** number by using the steps previously described. *This number is valid.*

15. Enter *073223* as the **STATE LICENSE** number.

16. Enter *073223* as the prescriber's **MEDICAID** number.

17. Ensure that the **COVERED BY MEDICAID** check box is checked if the prescriber is authorized to write prescriptions for Medicaid-supported patients.

Dr. Peterson is authorized to write prescriptions
for Medicaid-supported patients.

Community Pharmacy Practice

18. Click on the arrow to the right of the **Hospital** field.

Select *CITY HOSPITAL*.

19. Click on the arrow to the right of the **Status** field.

Select *Active* from the drop-down list to indicate that
the prescriber is in active practicing status.

20. Click on the **Save** 💾 icon located at the top right of the dialog box toolbar.

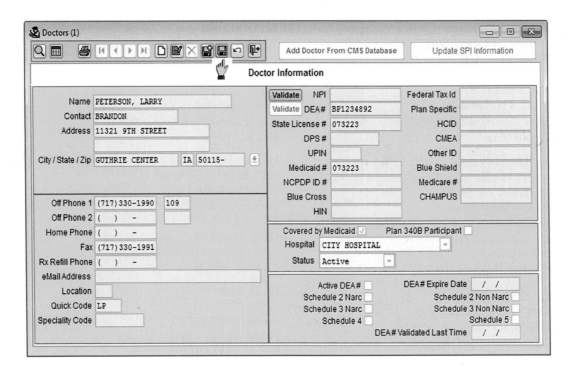

21. Print the screen by using the **Prnt Scrn** option on your keyboard. Press the **Prnt Scrn** key, open a blank Word document, **right click** the blank Word document, and then select **Paste**.

22. Check with your instructor on the preferred method for submitting your work.

23. Click on the **Close** 🚪 icon located at the top right of the dialog box toolbar.

EXERCISE

Practice using the software data entry skills by entering the following prescriber information. Follow Steps 1 through 23 for each prescriber who is added to the database. **Note:** If you check the DEA number and find it to be invalid, then note the reason (math calculation or initials) on your printout, and continue to enter the prescriber information.

Once entered, have another student check your data entry and math calculations of the DEA number verification, and submit your work when completed.

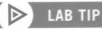 **LAB TIP**

In a commercial system, users would be able to validate DEA numbers within the application. This functionality has been removed for the educational version, which does not use assigned DEA numbers.

Prescriber Information

Dr. Catelynn Judith
9608 Barroll Lane, Suite 333
Kensington, MD 20895
Phone: 301-962-3140
Fax: 301-962-3144
DEA: AJ1256949-012
State License/Medicaid: 077332
Contact: Jen

Dr. Emma Francis
2208 Colonial Acres Court, Suite 444
Herndon, VA 20170
Phone: 703-430-3814
Fax: 703-430-3813
DEA: BF2368529
State License/Medicaid: 023569
Contact: Office Secretary

Dr. Markus Wayne
1812 Lincoln Highway, #52
Reston, VA 20190
Phone: 703-829-1100
Fax: 703-829-1111
DEA: AW7899567-134
State License/Medicaid: 096587
Contact: Judy

Dr. Jennifer Suz
1800 Lincoln Highway
Reston, VA 20194-1215
Phone: 703-829-1000
Fax: 703-829-1100
DEA: AS5478549
State License/Medicaid: 056921
Contact: Joe

Dr. Jacob Field
7500 Evans Street
Sterling, VA 20197
Phone: 703-571-2344
Fax: 703-571-2345
DEA: BF8527414
State License/Medicaid: 098632
Contact: Ralph, assistant

Dr. Lucille Moore
7500 Evans Street
Pittsburgh, PA 15218
Phone: 412-571-2300
Fax: 412-571-2301
DEA: AM5698521
State License/Medicaid: 000234
Contact: none

Dr. Tom Pane
5121 Brightwood Road, #110
Bethel Park, PA 15102
Phone: 412-835-4700
Fax: 412-835-4701
DEA: AP6985216
State License/Medicaid: 045698
Contact: Brenda

Dr. D. Kraft
11818 "F" Street
Omaha, NE 68137
Phone: 402-899-9911
Fax: 402-891-9912
DEA: AK2566327
State License/Medicaid: 023695
Contact: Brecken

Dr. I. Audubon
109 Eastside Drive
Omaha, NE 68137
Phone: 402-891-5521
Fax: 402-891-5522
DEA: AA7856416
State License/Medicaid: 030256
Contact: Office nurse

Enter a new Prescriber of your choosing.
Prescriber name:
Prescriber address:
Phone:
Fax:
DEA:
State License/Medicaid:
Contact:

Community Pharmacy Practice

LAB 2

Adding a New Patient to the Database in the Community Setting

■ Introduction

Pharmacy technicians work in a variety of practice settings. There are two primary areas, and one of them is commonly referred to as *community*. These stores can be owned by a single person or a group of persons (independent) or they can be part of a chain or franchise (e.g., CVS Pharmacy). Often, this type of store is also called *retail*, and most of the customers are ambulatory. This means that you will perform data entry and process prescriptions that have been brought in by hand, called or faxed in, or sent through electronic means, known as *e-prescribe*.

You will first enter information into a patient's profile and then process a variety of different medications by individually counting or preparing them. You may also have to answer questions regarding *over-the-counter* (OTC) medications, as well as durable and nondurable equipment. Examples of OTC medications include cough syrup, wound care supplies, vitamins, and herbal agents. Equipment could include diabetic meters and supplies, crutches, or prosthetic devices. In addition, there will be direct customer service and communication with other medical providers or insurance companies to process insurance online, known as *adjudication*. Technicians also use a cash register and will complete customer transactions, including cash payments.

> **MEDICATION SAFETY CONSIDERATION**
>
> Always ask **open-ended** questions, which require a response other than a **yes** or **no**. For example ask, "What is your birth date?" instead of, "Is your birth date May 26, 1927?" This requires the customer to stop and think about the question and form the answer, which can avoid mistakes if he or she is busy or gets distracted.

■ Lab Objectives

In this Lab, you will:

- Demonstrate the ability to enter correct medication and patient information into a profile while adhering to safety and confidentiality protocols.
- Demonstrate the ability to work in teams, and verify each other's work (simulate tech-check-tech [TCT]) when verifying patient information entered into the database profile.
- Practice patient data entry for a prescription that is brought in by hand, telephoned or faxed in, or electronically submitted.

ASHP goals: 3, 8, 12, 17, 18, 35, 36, and 41.

■ Scenario

Today, you are working in a simulated retail setting and learning to add new patients to the database.

■ Pre Lab Information

The Lab exercise will teach you how to perform the steps of entering a new customer or patient, and then you will be given several additional customers or patients to enter in the exercise. Ask another student to check your patient profile, and make any corrections before completing the assignments. You must enter all of the information listed to ensure that future prescriptions you enter will have complete information for each patient.

■ **Student Directions**

Estimated completion time: 30 minutes

1. Read through the steps in the Lab before performing the Lab exercise.
2. After reading through the Lab, perform the required steps to enter patient information.
3. Complete the exercise at the end of the Lab.

STEPS TO ADD A NEW PATIENT TO THE DATABASE

1. Access the main screen of Visual SuperScript.

2. Click on the **CUSTOMERS** button located on the left side of the screen. A dialog box entitled *Customers* will pop up.

3. Click on the **FIND** icon located on the dialog box toolbar. A dialog box entitled *Customer Lookup* will pop up.

4. Search the database to ensure that the patient is not already entered.

Type She to check for patient Mary Shedlock.

Note: No patient with a last name beginning with *She* will be found, and the *Customer Not Found* dialog box will pop up.

5. Within the *Customer Not Found* dialog box, click **YES** to add the customer. You can also click on the **ADD** button at the bottom of the *Customer Lookup* dialog screen to begin entering the patient's information. The *Customers* dialog box will open; the form is now ready to enter new patient information.

 LAB TIP

You may click **ENTER** after typing in the first three letters of the patient's name instead of scrolling through the results.

---

6. Type the patient's name in the **NAME** field.

Enter Shedlock, Mary E. as the patient name.

 LAB TIP

The **NAME** is a required field and allows up to 30 characters. The recommended format is the last name followed by a comma, a single space, the first name, a single space, and the middle initial and period or middle name, if known.

To facilitate searching your database, following the recommended format for entering names is very important. **Last names are entered first.** Example: Johnson, Linda P.

---

7. Enter Mary's date of birth in the **BIRTHDATE** field.

Enter 03/03/1960.

 HINT

The format for entering birthdates into the database is mm/dd/yyyy. Example: 06/07/1964 (Do not enter as 6/7/1964.)

---

8. Enter the patient's initials into the **Q Codes** (Quick Codes) field.

 LAB TIP

Q Codes allow you to expedite the search for customers when filling prescriptions.

9. Click on the arrow located to the right of the **Pay Type** data entry field. Select the appropriate **Pay Type**.

Select Private. **Click OK.**

Note: Pay Type determines how prescriptions filled for this patient are priced and who is expected to pay for them. Two **Pay Types** are permissible: *Private* and *Insurance.*

 LAB TIP

Each patient profile should have some type of payment information, and this information can be recorded as either INSURANCE or CASH or both. Check with the patient each time a prescription is requested for filling; the information may have changed, or the patient may have new insurance. Checking will save time and additional work at pickup.

10. Click on the arrow located to the right of the **Gender** data entry field.

Select appropriate gender as *Female.* **Click OK.**

11. Next in the **Family** field, a pop-up dialog box asking, "Is Customer also head of family?" will appear. Click **No**. Enter *Matthew Shedlock* as the family head in the text box next to the **Family** icon. Press **Enter**. The *Family Head Not Found* dialog box will appear. Click **Yes** to add him as the family head.

Note: Family is a required field. Customers are grouped into families, with each family having one individual designated as the **Family Head**. Each customer is linked to the family database by reference to the **Family Head**.

 HINT

The abbreviation *HOH* stands for *Head of Household*, which indicates the family head.

12. The *Families* dialog box will appear. Enter the address and telephone number information. Once the following information is entered, **Save** 🖫 and **Close** 🗗 out of *Families*.

Enter *1386 Quincy Lane, Allston, MA 02134. 703-464-0100.*

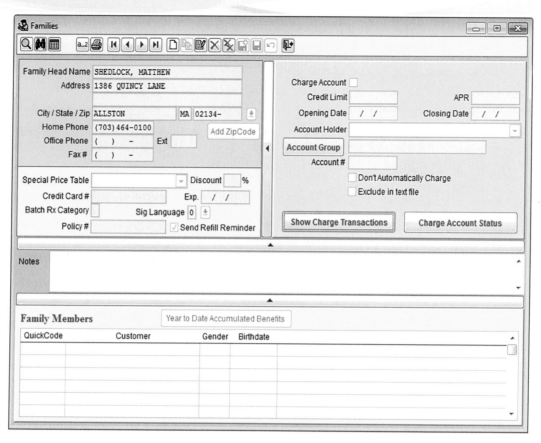

13. In the **NOTES** field , enter the following information.

Patient is hard of hearing in left ear.

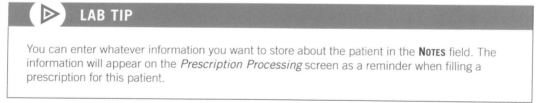

LAB TIP

You can enter whatever information you want to store about the patient in the **NOTES** field. The information will appear on the *Prescription Processing* screen as a reminder when filling a prescription for this patient.

14. In the **PATIENT ID TYPE** field, check that **DRIVER LICENSE** is selected. If not, enter the following:

057915228

15. Tab to the **RX ELIGIBILITY** field, and select *Dependent Parent* from the drop-down menu. Click **OK**.

16. In the **PLACE OF SERVICE** field, ensure that Pharmacy is selected.

17. In **PATIENT RESIDENCE** field, ensure that Home is selected.

18. Tab to the **CHILDPROOF OPTION** field. By default, this box will be **CP** for every customer that is added to the database.

Leave the default CP setting for Mary.

LAB TIP

The Poison and Prevention Packaging ACT of 1970 requires the use of a child-proof lid unless otherwise specified. If a customer desires easy-open lids, then use the drop-down menu and indicate this here.

19. Tab to the **No of Labels** field. Indicate a *1* in this field unless the patient requests two labels at the time the prescription for this patient is filled.

Mary only needs one label right now.

MEDICATION SAFETY CONSIDERATION

Always ask about allergies on **every** prescription fill. Allergies can change daily and can cause harm or even death to a patient if a medication interacts with another.

20. Click on the **Allergies** tab located on the bottom half of the *Customers* form.

21. Click on the **New** 🗋 icon located on the bottom right of the Customers form. An *Allergen Lookup* table pops up.

22. Key in the first three letters of the allergy in the **Allergy** data entry field. Use the scroll bar to select the appropriate allergy. Select the appropriate allergy by clicking on the allergy, and then click **OK**.

Key in MOR. Select morphine. Click OK.

23. Click on the **Other Drugs** tab.

24. Click on the **New** 🗋 icon located on the bottom right of the *Customers* form. Press the **Enter** key to access a list of drugs. A *Drug Name Lookup* table pops up.

MEDICATION SAFETY CONSIDERATION

The **Other Drugs** grid contains information about other drugs that the patient is currently taking. These prescription drugs may have been purchased from a different pharmacy, or they may be over-the-counter (OTC), herbals, or vitamins. For each such drug, a start date and estimated days of supply may also be entered. The purpose of recording this information is to check for possible drug interactions and duplicate ingredients and therapy, no matter where they were purchased.

25. Type the name of the drug in the *Name* dialog box to look up the drug. Click the desired drug to select it. Click **OK**.

Mary Shedlock began taking Vitamin E 400 soft-gel qd in 12/2006.

26. Click the **Disease Profile** tab.

27. Click on the **New** 🗋 icon located on the bottom right of the *Customers* form. A red bar appears across the *Disease Profile* table. Click inside the *Disease Profile* to turn it blue, which indicates the information can now be entered.

Note: The **Disease Profile** grid contains a list of diseases for which the customer has been diagnosed. The information contained in this grid is used to check for drug-disease contraindications each time a prescription is filled for the patient.

28. Click the **F2** function key, and a *CDIAGCODE* table pops up. Look up the disease by typing the first few letters of the name of the disease. Click the desired disease to select it. Click **OK**.

Enter diabetes mellitus for the disease.

Choose **DIABETES MELLITUS** (Diagnosis Code 208).

29. Click on the **SAVE** 💾 icon located at the top right of the toolbar in the *Customers* dialog box.

30. Print the screen by using the **PRNT SCRN** option on your keyboard: Press the **PRNT SCRN** key, open a blank Word document, **RIGHT CLICK** the blank Word document, and then select **PASTE**.

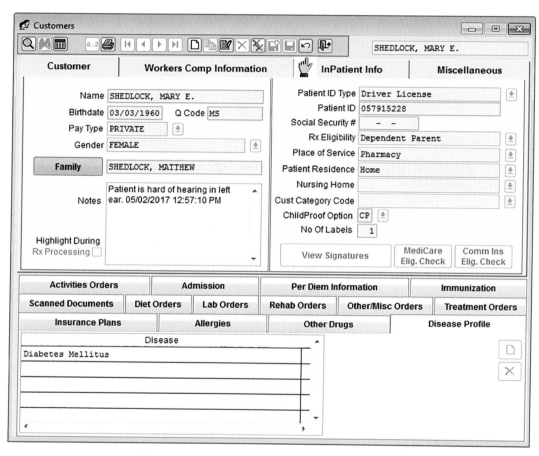

31. Click on the **CLOSE** 🚪 icon located at the top right of the toolbar.

EXERCISE

Enter the following customers into the database using the information provided. Refer back to Lab 1 if any Zip codes are not entered into the database. Have a fellow technician student check your profiles (on your computer) for data entry errors. Correct all errors if any are found by using the editing function.

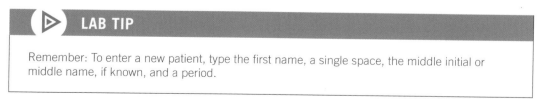

▷ **LAB TIP**

Remember: To enter a new patient, type the first name, a single space, the middle initial or middle name, if known, and a period.

Note: Unless indicated, **Rx Eligibility** will be the default **Not Specified**; **Place of Service** will be **Pharmacy**; and **Residence** will be **Home**.

Patient and HOH: Ray Ruhl
DOB: 2/21/57
SSN: 472-97-4562
Allergies: penicillin (PCN)
170 Laurel Way
Herndon, VA 20170
Home phone: 703-481-5200
DL: 548492721
Pay type: Private
Requests easy-open caps
No known allergies
Other medications: albuterol inhaler 90 mcg
    (package size 8.500), Singulair 10 mg tablet
Disease state: Asthma (Diagnosis Code 493)

Patient and HOH: Robert Gamble
DOB: 3/15/57
SSN: 423-11-3333
Allergies: PCN
1447 Woodbrook Court
Reston, VA 20194-1215
Home phone: 703-787-9000
Pay type: Private
Hospice patient
Requests easy-open lids
Disease state: Leukemia of unspecified cell type
    (Diagnosis Code 208)
Other medications: Colace 100 mg capsule

Patient: Julie Douglas
HOH: Doug Douglas (same address as Julie)
DOB: 8/14/77
Pay type: Private
Allergies: codeine
Not pregnant
SSN: 333-56-9887
12124 Walnut Branch Road
Audubon, IA 50025
Home phone: 571-203-0000
Notes: Deliver prescriptions to home address
    before 5:00 PM

Patient: Katherine Cald
HOH: Timothy Cald (same address as Katherine)
DOB: 3/20/57
DL# I4569821
Allergies: cephalosporins
Insurance plan: Anthem 1
11200 Longwood Grove
Elk Horn, IA 51531
Home phone: 703-464-1700

Patient and HOH: Annette Mang
DOB: 1/12/57
SSN: 362-89-5663
Allergies: morphine
1490 Autumn Ridge Court
Reston, VA 20194-1215
Home phone: 703-834-0500
Pay type: Private
Other medications: alprazolam 1 mg tablet,
    Seroquel 25 mg tablet
Wants duplicate labels

Patient and HOH: Dana Walks
DOB: 4/21/57
Allergies: PCN
1206 Weatherstone Court
Ralston, NE 68128
Home phone: 703-430-6300
Pay type: Private
Requests easy-open caps
Notes: Has not signed HIPAA form
Other medications: Skelaxin 800 mg tablet PRN,
    spironolactone 100 mg tablet

Patient and HOH: Martin Marin
DOB: 5/17/50
Allergies: No known allergies (NKA)
11324 Olde Tiverton Circle
Ralston, NE 68128
Home phone: 703-437-5000
Other medications: Aldactone 100 mg tablet,
    Serevent Diskus 50 mcg inhaler
Would like two labels
Would like easy-open caps
Work-related injury
Contact at work: Steve Thomas, Manager
Bonds, Inc., 309 Third Street, Fister, NE 68110
Work phone: 402-698-2356

Enter yourself as a patient using similar information listed in each category previously used. This will allow future assignments to be completed using yourself as a patient.

 LAB TIP

To go back and check each other's work and look up your patient, use the vertical scroll bar located on the right side of the pop-up dialog box to view customer information. To facilitate searching your database: **Remember: Search using the first three letters of the last name ONLY.**

LAB 3

Making a Change to the Patient Profile or Prescriber Information

■ Introduction

Working in a community or retail setting, patients will come to the pharmacy on a regular or monthly cycle for their *maintenance medications*. These medications are typically refilled, based on cyclic laboratory work, and they do not change much. For example, a patient who has a diagnosis of high blood pressure is prescribed lisinopril 10 mg; unless blood work indicates a significant change, this prescription will be rewritten or (refilled) every 3 to 6 months. The new prescription may be called in, sent electronically, or brought in by the patient after his or her appointment.

Other types of medications, such as cold, allergy, or antibiotic medications for an acquired infection, may be needed periodically in addition to their regular medications.

MEDICATION SAFETY CONSIDERATION

Updating and inputting the correct information for a new prescription is extremely important as the patient may have an existing medication that may interact with the new order. In addition, always ask about allergies on every visit. A patient may have developed something new since the last visit, and it needs to be on his or her profile.

In addition to prescription medications, a physician may order specific over-the-counter (OTC) medications or vitamins or herbals. Examples are fish oil, baby aspirin, and vitamin E. Although the patient can purchase these items from the shelves in the OTC area, once an OTC medication is brought to the counter, you should enter this information in the profile as a new drug. Changes to the profile need to be maintained and kept up to date to ensure that ALL of the medications that are being taken and the correct provider information are reviewed and maintained in the patient profile.

■ Lab Objectives

In this Lab, you will:

- Demonstrate how to identify information required for updating patient profiles.
- Demonstrate how to edit prescriber information.
- Perform the steps to review and add or edit patient information in a profile.

■ Scenario

You are working in the simulated retail pharmacy today, and you have been presented with new information that needs to be added or edited on a patient or physician's profile.

■ Pre Lab Information

Review Labs 1 and 2 for the steps for entering physician and patient information into the database. Remember to look up (**SEARCH**) a patient or physician using the **last three letters** only.

■ **Student Directions**

Estimated completion time: 30 minutes

1. Read through the steps in the Lab before performing the Lab exercise.
2. After reading through the Lab, perform the required steps to edit or add information.
3. Complete the exercise at the end of the Lab.

STEPS TO CHANGE THE PATIENT PROFILE OR PRESCRIBER INFORMATION

1. Access the main screen of Visual SuperScript.

2. Click on the **CUSTOMERS** button located on the left side of the screen. A dialog box entitled *Customers* will pop up.

3. Click on the **FIND** icon, which is located on the top left of the *Customers* dialog box toolbar.

4. A dialog box entitled *Customer Lookup* will pop up. Enter the first three letters of the customer's last name into the **NAME** data entry field. Click on the patient name for whom information will be updated.

Find John M. Smith.

5. The selected customer name is highlighted in blue. Click on the **EDIT** 📝 icon located at the bottom of the *Customer Lookup* dialog box. A dialog box entitled *Customers* will pop up.

6. Click on the **EDIT** 📝 icon located in the middle of the *Customers* toolbar at the top of the dialog box.

7. Tab to the desired data entry field, and key in the appropriate changes.

Change John M. Smith's DOB to *02/22/1947*.

> ▷ **LAB TIP**
>
> Deleting the existing information before adding the new information is not necessary. Simply key the new information into the highlighted data entry field.

8. Click on the **SAVE** 💾 icon located on the toolbar at the top right of the *Customers* dialog box.

9. Click on the **CLOSE** 🚪 icon located on the toolbar at the top right of the *Customers* dialog box. The edited information has now been added to the database.

10. Make note of the updated information in the *Customer Lookup* dialog box. Click **OK** at the bottom of the *Customer Lookup* dialog box.

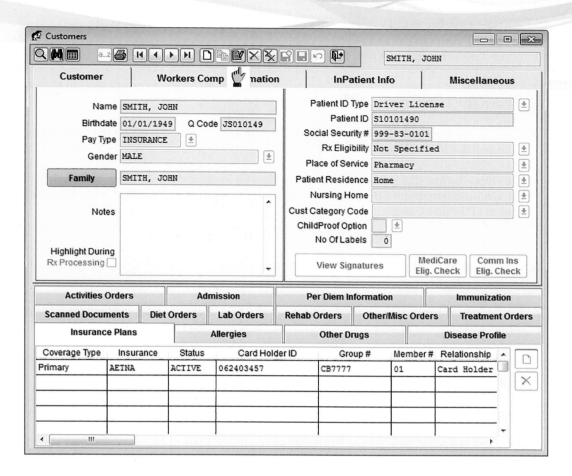

11. Ask another student to check your work to verify that the information has changed in your computer.

12. Print the screen by using the **PRNT SCRN** option on your keyboard. Press the **PRNT SCRN** key, open a blank Word document, **RIGHT CLICK** the blank Word document, and then select **PASTE**.

EXERCISE

Practice using the software data entry skills by entering the following patient information. Submit work as previously described (**PRNT SCRN**) when completed.

Change the following patient information:
- Jada Sanchez's birthday is 08/30/1996, and she has a new allergy for penicillin (PCN).
- Margaret Pena is the HOH, and her home phone number is 555-639-5489.

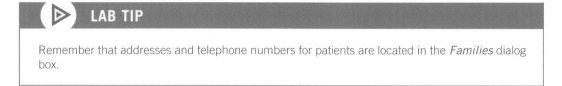

LAB TIP

Remember that addresses and telephone numbers for patients are located in the *Families* dialog box.

1. Access the main screen of Visual SuperScript.

2. Click on the **Doctors** button located on the left side of the screen. A dialog box entitled *Doctors* will pop up.

3. Click on the **Find** 🔍 icon located on the toolbar at the top of the dialog box. The *Doctor Lookup* dialog box will appear.

4. The *Doctor Lookup* dialog box offers several choices for locating the prescriber's records. Key in the first three letters of the prescriber's last name in the **Name** data entry field. Click **OK** at the bottom of the dialog box.

Key in BOS for Dr. Robert Bosworth.

5. Click on the **Edit** 📝 icon located on the toolbar at the top of the form. The form is now ready for you to edit the prescriber information.

6. Tab through the form to reach the desired data entry field. Make the appropriate changes to the form.

Enter the office phone 2 extension of 104.

7. Click on the **Save** 💾 icon located at the top right of the toolbar.

8. Print the screen by using the **Prnt Scrn** option on your keyboard. Press the **Prnt Scrn** key, open a blank Word document, **Right Click** the blank Word document, and then select **Paste**.

QUICK CHALLENGE

Scenario

Dr. Karen Davis is a prescribing physician in your area. She has recently married and changed her last name to a hyphenated name, Dr. Karen Davis-Bendfeldt. The managing pharmacist has asked you to update Dr. Davis-Bendfeldt's records.

Task

Following the steps from the exercise entitled, *Steps to Edit a Prescriber's Information*, edit Dr. Karen Davis-Bendfeldt's information. Print or save the form, and submit it for verification.

LAB 4

Adding Third-Party Payment Information to the Database and Reviewing Patient Plan Information

■ Introduction

When working in a community setting, insurance processing and billing command much of the prescription process and daily tasks. Technicians must understand how to communicate with third-party companies, as well as customers, and to identify the needed information to process medication claims online (adjudication).

Knowing generic and brand names, following formulary requirements, and entering the information into the database for each patient are also daily tasks. Knowing how insurance cards are laid out and correctly entering information are required to prevent rejections. Other types of payment such as Medicaid, Medicare, workers compensation, and TRICARE (Veteran's Administration) also have specific requirements to process a medication claim.

■ Lab Objectives

In this Lab, you will:

- Add a new insurance plan to the database.
- Enter information regarding insurance billing procedures.
- Identify and enter key features of a sample insurance card required for patient profile.

■ Scenario

Today, you are working with third-party companies and other plans, as well as reviewing cards for patients already in the database system. You will review sample cards and identify key information required to be in the database system. You will then enter a specific insurance plan and all the components required in the database for your pharmacy.

■ Pre Lab Information

First, you will see a series a different samples of insurance cards to identify the key components, which will help you become familiar with the types commonly seen in a community practice as a technician. Answer any questions related to each card.

Next, you will complete an exercise to enter an insurance (third-party) plan into the database. Using the knowledge gained from your review of the cards, you can now identify the required information for a particular plan.

 LAB TIP

The insurance plan name could be the same name as the insurance company. However, both restrictions and copay requirements may be different, and they may also need to be submitted with different biller identification numbers (BINs) and/or PROCESSOR CONTROL numbers. **Therefore it is best to avoid associating the names of insurance plans with the names of insurance companies.**

Similarly, there are Pharmacy Benefits Managers, who are not an INSURANCE COMPANY. Rather, a Pharmacy Benefits Manager is a clearing house for the online (adjudication) process in a pharmacy, such as ARGUS Health Systems and Diversified Pharmacy Services (DPS); consequently, it is best to avoid associating the names of insurance plans with the names of these processors as well.

Most often, each insurance plan that requires a unique combination of BIN and PROCESSOR CONTROL numbers should have a separate name and a separate record.

- The group number and member identification (ID) are specific for each patient and are required to be in the patient's profile.
- Person code, date of birth, and sex code are also required to be in the patient's profile for processing a medication payment.

 LAB TIP

The primary covered person is coded 1, the spouse is coded 2, and children follow in sequential order.

- Other information that will be useful is the copay amounts for medications, based on the company's formulary. Each insurance plan is different, and this information will usually be on the card. For example; below the prescription drug is 10/20/40, which indicates a $10, $20, or $40 copay amount, depending on the drug's place in the formulary. For example, a generic drug is less expensive than a brand-name medication and is usually the lowest copay available.

■ Student Directions

Estimated completion time: 45 minutes

1. Read through the steps in the Lab before performing the Lab exercise.
2. After reading through the Lab, perform the required steps listed in the Lab.
3. Answer the questions at the end of the Lab.
4. Complete the exercise at the end of the Lab.

STEPS TO ADD INSURANCE PLANS TO THE DATABASE

1. Access the main screen of Visual SuperScript.

2. Click on the **INSURANCE PLANS** button located on the left side of the screen. A dialog box entitled *Insurance Plans* will appear.

   Note: The *Insurance Plans* form is used to maintain a database of insurance plans to which your customers subscribe. The *Insurance Plans* form contains three tabs. Be sure the **INSURANCE PLAN DATA** tab is open when following these steps.

3. Click on the **NEW** 🗋 icon located on the toolbar at the top of the *Insurance Plans* dialog box. The *Insurance Plan Lookup* dialog box will appear.

4. Enter the name of the insurance plan you want to add in the **PLAN NAME** data entry field.

   Enter *COSPLS* as the plan name.

   Note: This plan does not exist. Click **ADD PLAN** at the bottom of the *Insurance Plan Lookup* dialog box and a form prepopulates for AARP.

5. In the **PLAN NAME** data entry field, replace *AARP* with *COSPLS*. Skip the **LONG NAME** data entry field. This field is not editable. Tab to the **COMPANY** data entry field, and click on the arrow to access the drop-down menu. Type in the first three letters of the company name. A list of names will then pop up from which you can select the company name.

Choose *Hold RX* as the company name, and click OK.

 LAB TIP

6. Tab to the next data entry field underneath *Company Phone*. This field is used to identify the pharmacy to the insurance company for billing purposes. Click on the arrow located to the right of the data entry field. Scroll through the drop-down menu, and select the desired **IDENTIFICATION QUALIFIER** by clicking on the name.

Choose *NCPDP Provider ID* as the identification qualifier.

7. Tab to the next unnamed data entry field. Enter the pharmacy ID number in the next data entry field.

Enter *6503829* as the pharmacy ID.

Note: In most cases, the unique pharmacy ID number is the National Association Board of Pharmacy (NABP) number.

8. Tab to the **BILLING METHOD** data entry field. Click the arrow located to the right of the **BILLING METHOD** data entry field. Choose the desired **BILLING METHOD** by clicking on the desired choice in the drop-down menu.

Choose *Electronic Billing* as the billing method.

9. Tab to the **MAX DAYS FOR REFILLS** data entry field.

Note: This data entry field specifies the period during which prescriptions must be refilled to be eligible for reimbursement under this plan.

Enter *365* as the **MAX DAYS FOR REFILLS**.

10. Tab to the **MAX REFILLS** data entry field.

Enter *6* as the **MAX REFILLS**.

Note: This data entry field represents the number of times the insurance company will pay on a given prescription to be refilled. A value of zero (0) implies that refills are not allowed.

11. Tab to the **MAX DAYS SUPPLY** data entry field.

Note: This data entry field represents a payer-imposed limit, if any, on the amount of a medication that may be dispensed at a time.

Enter *32* as the **MAX DAYS SUPPLY**.

12. Check the **ADD SALES TAX** check box if your state imposes a sales tax on medicines. The sales tax will then be billed to the insurance company.

13. The **DIS GEN UNLESS DAW** box will be checked for insurance companies that require generic drugs to be dispensed unless the prescriber specifies dispense as written (DAW) on the prescription.

Check this box.

14. Check the **OTC COVERED** box if over-the-counter (OTC) drugs are covered under this insurance plan.

OTC drugs are covered under this plan.

15. **Cost Pref #1**, **#2**, and **#3** (cost preferences) are the three choices for calculating the ingredient cost of the drug. For each preference, the available choices are displayed in a drop-down menu. Click the arrow to the right of the data entry field to access the list. Select the three cost preferences. When pricing a prescription, Visual SuperScript first attempts to calculate the ingredient cost based on **Cost Pref #1**. If **Cost Pref #1** is unavailable (as indicated by a zero in that field in the drug record), then Visual SuperScript uses **Cost Pref #2**, and so on.

Enter *AWP* (average wholesale price) as **Cost Pref #1**.

Enter *MAC* (manufacturers' average cost) as **Cost Pref #2**.

Enter *Direct* as **Cost Pref #3**.

16. Tab to the **Usual & Cust Charges?** data entry field. Click on the arrow located to the right of the data entry field. Four options are provided on a drop-down list. Click on the desired name from the drop-down list.

Select *All Drugs* from the list.

Note: The **Usual & Cust Charges?** data entry field indicates whether the insurance company requires you to submit the usual and customary charges if the pharmacy's price of the medication is lower than the price based on the ingredient cost–plus–dispensing fee formula specified by the insurance company.

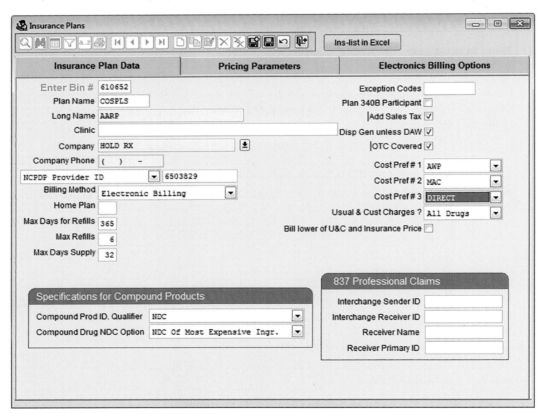

17. Click on the dark pink tab entitled *Pricing Parameters*. The *Pricing Parameters* form will be active and ready for data entry.

18. Key in the desired markup factor in the **Brand Markup** data entry field.

Note: The **Brand Markup** is the factor by which the AWP (or the MAC or direct cost) of the drug is multiplied to arrive at the ingredient cost of the drug for billing purposes. For example, a 10% markup should be entered as 1.1. A 100% markup should be entered as 2.00.

Enter *1* as the **Brand Markup**.

19. Key in the **BRAND DISP FEE** allowed by the insurance company.

Enter 3.50 as the Brand Disp Fee.

Note: The **BRAND DISP FEE** data entry field contains the dispensing fee allowed by the insurance company for brand-name drugs. The dispensing fee is added to the ingredient cost to arrive at the price of the drug.

20. Key in the markup factor for brand-name OTC drugs in the **BRAND MARKUP FOR OTC** data entry field.

Enter 1.25 as the Brand Markup for an OTC Drug.

21. Key in the amount of money to be paid by the customer (copay) for each brand-name prescription in the **BRAND COPAY** data entry field.

Enter 20 as the Brand Copay.

Note: The pharmacy collects the copay amount from the customer at the time the prescription is picked up from the pharmacy.

22. Check the **IS IT PERCENT?** box if the figure entered in the copay data entry field is to be treated as a percentage of the price rather than an absolute dollar amount. For example, if the price of the drug is $45.00, an entry of 10 is in the copay field, and the **IS IT PERCENT?** box is not checked, then the copay computed by the system would be a $10.00 flat copay fee. However, if the **IS IT PERCENT?** box is checked, then the copay will be computed as $4.50 (10% of $45.00).

Leave the Is It Percent? box unchecked.

23. The **BRAND DISCOUNTED COPAY** data entry field should reflect the same copay as the corresponding **BRAND COPAY** field *unless* your pharmacy has decided to offer a lower copay amount than is required by the insurance company.

Key in the correct Brand Discount Copay as 20,
and leave the Is It Percent? information blank.

24. Key in the required information in the second column of the *Pricing Parameters* form. The second column is entitled **GENERIC**.

Generic Markup: 1

Generic Disp. Fee: $3.50

Generic Markup for OTC: $1.25

Generic Copay: $5

Generic Is It Percent? No

Generic Discounted Copay: $5

Generic Is It Percent? No

25. Tab to the **SAME COPAY AS GENERICS FOR BRAND DRUGS WITH NO GEN** data entry field. Check this box if the copay amounts for brand-name and generic drugs are different and the insurance company allows the customer to pay the same copay for a generic drug as it does for a brand-name drug that has no generic drug available.

Check the Same Copay as Generics box.

Note: Usually, lower copay amounts are required for generic drugs versus brand-name drugs as an incentive for patients to choose generic over brand-name drugs. Under some plans, the customer is allowed to pay the lower copay amount when a drug has no generic drug available.

26. Tab to the **Max Payment for an Rx** data entry field. This field specifies the maximum amount the insurance company will pay for a single prescription.

Enter a large value such as 9999 if no limit exists.

27. The **Perc. of Cost Diff. Between Brand & Generics Paid** data entry field specifies the *percentage* of the difference between the price of the brand-name drug and the price of the generic drug that the insurance company requires the patient to pay if the patient chooses a brand name over the generic drug. Enter the correct percentage difference in the **Perc. of Cost Diff. Between Brand & Generics Paid** field.

Enter 80 as the percentage of cost difference.

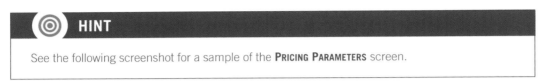

See the following screenshot for a sample of the **Pricing Parameters** screen.

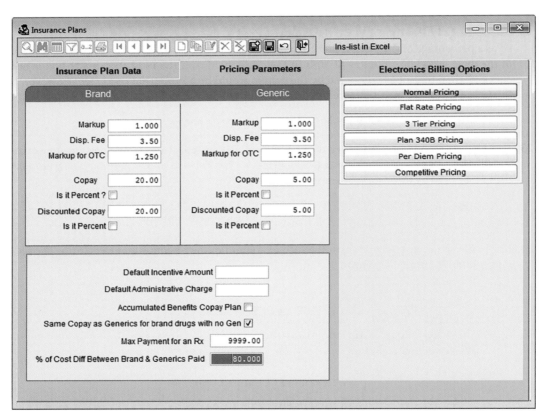

28. Click on the **Electronic Billing Options** tab. The *Electronic Billing Options* form is active and ready for data entry.

Note: The information contained in the **Electronic Billing Options** form determines to whom claims are sent for adjudication, as well as the format in which they are sent. Successful adjudication requires that all items be entered as completely and accurately as possible.

29. The **El. Biller** (electronic biller) data entry field specifies the company to which the electronic claim is initially delivered. Click on the arrow located to the right of the **El. Biller** data entry field. A dialog box entitled *Insurance Carrier* pops up. Type the first three letters of the insurance company (in this case, *Nat*). Select *NATL. DATA CORP.* Then click **OK**.

30. The **BIN** identifies the party to whom the electronic biller (from step 29) needs to forward the claim. This field is required for all electronically transmitted plans. Most insurance companies will list the **BIN** on the insurance card issued to the customer. The **BIN** always consists of six numeric characters. Key in the correct **BIN**.

Enter 510455 as the BIN.

31. The **Proc. Ctrl.** (processing control number [PCS]) data entry field is a required field for all electronically transmitted plans. The PCS may also be referred to as the *Carrier ID*. Key in the appropriate *PCS* or *Carrier ID*.

Enter HCS as the PCS or Carrier ID.

32. Tab to the **Required Prescriber ID** (required medical physician [MD] or prescriber ID number) data entry field. Click on the arrow located to the right of the data entry field. Select and click on the appropriate type of ID number that the insurance company uses to identify the prescriber. For successful adjudication, selecting the appropriate identifier for each specific plan is imperative.

Select DEA# as the identifier.

33. Click on the arrow located to the right of the **Default Other Coverage Code** data entry field. Click on the appropriate coverage code from the table in the *Default Other Coverage Code* dialog box. Click **OK** located at the bottom of the dialog box.

Select 0—Not Specified as the code.

34. Click on the arrow located to the right of the **Default Oth Code for Secondary Billing** data entry field. Click on the appropriate coverage code from the table in the *Default Other Coverage Code* dialog box. Click **OK** located at the bottom of the dialog box.

Select 0—Not Specified as the code.

35. Click on the arrow located to the right of the **Default Rx Origin Code** data entry field. Indicate if the third-party payer (e.g., insurance company) requires prescriptions to be written (select *1—Written Prescription*) or if the third-party payer has no preference on the form or origin of the prescription (select *0—Not Specified*). After choosing the correct prescription origin code, click **OK** located at the bottom of the *Rx Origin Code* dialog box.

Select 0—Not Specified as the code.

36. Click on the arrow located on the right side of the **Default Rx Elig Clar Code** data entry field. Select the correct prescription eligibility clarification code from the table in the dialog box. Click **OK** located on the bottom of the *Rx Elig Clar Code* dialog box.

Select 1—No Override as the code.

37. Beneath the **Default Customer Residence Code** data entry field, check the **Medicaid** box.

38. The check boxes located on the right side of the *Electronic Billing Options* form are optional data entry fields. Completion of these fields may be required for some insurance plans. To ensure proper adjudication of your claims, a phone call to the insurance company's help desk may be necessary to find out which data entry fields are required. Check the appropriate boxes.

Check the XMIT Multiple Claims (transmit multiple claims) check box to allow for transmitting multiple claims in a single transaction. If this check box is not checked, then claims will be transmitted one at a time.

39. Click on the **Save** [💾] icon located at the top of the *Insurance Plans* form. The insurance plan has now been added to the database.

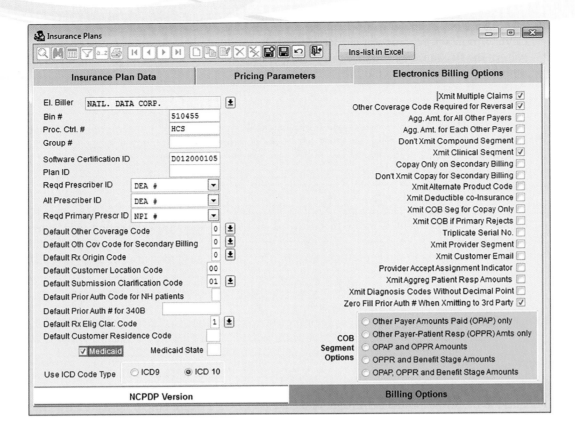

40. Print the screen by using the **Prnt Scrn** option on your keyboard. Press the **Prnt Scrn** key, open a blank Word document, **Right Click** the blank Word document, and then select **Paste**.

QUESTIONS FOR REVIEW

1. _____ Associating the name of an insurance plan with the name of the insurance company is best.
   a. True
   b. False

2. _____ A pharmacy benefits manager is the person who may process insurance claims for the insurance company.
   a. True
   b. False

3. The three tab names on the *Insurance Plans* form are:

   (1) _____

   (2) _____

   (3) _____

4. _____ The **Identification Qualifier** is:
   a. A coded number that identifies the insurance company
   b. Used to identify the prescriber for third-party billing
   c. The same for every plan
   d. An optional data entry field

5. _____ **BILLING METHOD** choices include:
   a. Electronic billing
   b. Universal claim form
   c. Fax
   d. Both a and b

6. _____ The **MAX REFILLS** data entry field represents the:
   a. Maximum number of refills the pharmacy will allow the patient to have
   b. Maximum number of refills the insurance plan will allow the patient to have
   c. Number of times the insurance company will pay on a given prescription to be refilled
   d. Maximum number of refills the prescriber will allow the patient to have

7. _____ Does your state impose a sales tax on prescription medications?
   a. Yes
   b. No

8. _____ The copay amount for brand-name medications should always be marked as a percentage of the price of the medication.
   a. True
   b. False

9. _____ An example of a third-party payer is the patient's insurance company.
   a. True
   b. False

10. _____ The information contained in the *Electronic Billing Options* form determines:
    a. To whom claims are sent for adjudication
    b. The format in which claims are sent
    c. Both a and b.
    d. The patient copay amount only

11. _____ The *Electronic Billing Options* form will be active only if the billing method choice is electronic billing.
    a. True
    b. False

12. The PCN may also be referred to as the _____ or the _____.

13. _____ The BIN:
    a. Identifies the party to whom the electronic biller needs to forward the claim
    b. Is a required field for all electronically transmitted plans
    c. Is a six-digit number on the customer's insurance card
    d. Is all of the above

14. _____ NCPDP:
    a. Is the official standard for pharmacy claims in the Health Insurance Portability and Accountability Act (HIPAA)
    b. Is the National Council for Prescription Drug Programs
    c. Provides pharmacies with a unique identifying number for interactions with federal agencies and third-party processors
    d. Is all of the above

EXERCISE

Scenario

The pharmacy manager has asked you to update the database by adding a new insurance plan. Adding the new plan by the end of the day is important to submit a patient's prescription claim electronically. Your manager provides you with a detailing of the pricing information:

Pharmacy ID: 6503829

Brand markup is 1.5 (prescription and OTC)

The pharmacy offers a discount only for generic drug copay: 1%

Task

Use the following insurance plan information, as well as the information that the managing pharmacist has provided, to add an insurance plan to the database. Select *Not Specified* for any insurance information that is not provided. Submit each tabbed area of the *Insurance Plans* form on completion.

Insurance Plan Information

Plan Name: SureWay

Plan Details: The maximum number of refills allowed is 12. The maximum number of days' supply is 32. Refills are allowed for a maximum of 1 year. The pharmacy should always dispense generic medications unless otherwise indicated by the physician. If a generic medication is not available, then the customer will pay the generic copay amount for the brand-name medication. If a generic medication is available but the customer prefers the brand-name medication, then the customer must pay 90% of the price cost difference between the brand-name and generic drugs. All medications are subject to usual and customary charges. OTC drugs are not covered under this plan.

Company name: SystemED

ID qualifier: NCPDP—Format version 3A

Electronic biller: Pro-Serv

BIN: 610053

Processor control: 7Q 7700970

Cost preference: AWP

Dispensing fees: $3.00 brand name and generic

Flat copay amounts: $10.00 brand name; $2.50 generic

Maximum payment: None

Prescriber qualifier: DEA number

Note: A code is required for claim reversal.

Task

Answer the following questions using the provided figures.

HOPPER HEALTH

HOSPITAL ADMISSIONS REQUIRE PRIOR APPROVAL

GROUP NAME: ABC Industries
CARDHOLDER: JOHN DOE
RX BENEFIT: $15/30/75
YBC999999999 99

GROUP: 272550000001
BCBSKC RX   1-800-228-1436
BC PLAN: 240   BS PLAN: 740
CUST SERV: 816-232-8396/800-822-2583

75.00 EMER ROOM
20.00 OFFICE VISIT

Using the above figure, answer the following questions:

1. What is the group number for this patient? _____

2. Who is the owner of this card? _____

3. Furosemide and Mobic were prescribed for this patient and the plan formulary covers generic at the lowest copay amount.

   a. At what copay amount would Furosemide be charged? $_____

   b. At what copay amount would Mobic be charged? $_____

Complete Health Insurance

Cardholder: **JAKE SAMPLE**	For Pharmacy: **1-800-555-1234**
ID#: **ABC0000000000**	
Group#: **EFG0000000000**	For Patient: **1-800-555-5678**
Office visit copay: **$25.00**	
RX Benefit: **$10/20/40**	

Using the above figure, answer the following questions.

1. A prescription was written for Jake Sample for generic amoxicillin.

   a. Jake would be coded as what? _____

   b. What copay would be the charge for this prescription? $_____

   c. What coverage type does this patient have? _____

   d. There is a question concerning the prescription, and the pharmacist asks that you provide a phone number for a person to whom the question can be asked. What number would you provide the pharmacist?

   _____

EMP HealthyLife
Health Insurance

SUBSCRIBER NAME:
JOHN DOE

MEMBER ID #:
000000000A

GROUP #:
000000000B

COPAY
$20/40/60

COVERAGE TYPE
EMP

For pharmacy use: 1-800-555-1234
For patient use: 1-800-555-5678

Using the above figure, answer the following questions.

1. What is the member ID number for John Doe? _____

2. There is a rejection and question for coverage. What number would you as the technician need to call for verification?

_____

3. The patient is questioning the prescription written because it states "brand necessary." The best way to resolve this issue is to have the patient call the insurance company to discuss the requirements. What number would the patient need to call?

_____

LAB 5

Adding a Drug to the Database and Other Inventory Tasks

▪ Introduction

Since the establishment of the U.S. Food and Drug Administration (FDA) and then the designation of legend (prescription) and over-the-counter drugs, all medications sold on the market are required to meet certain criteria and receive approval. In 1972, The Drug Listing Act began the process of giving every drug a unique 10-digit code for identification. These numbers can be separated into sections and indicate the manufacturer, product code, and package code.

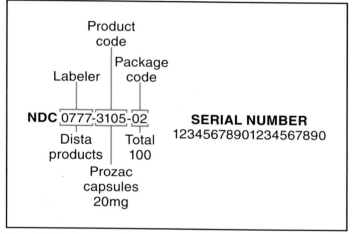

From *Mosby's pharmacy technician: principles and practice*, ed 4, St Louis, 2016, Mosby.

As a pharmacy technician, you will participate in inventory control and ordering on a daily basis. The task of processing a prescription requires data entry based on the specific drug ordered, including its brand or generic name and often the manufacturer if your pharmacy has a special wholesaler agreement. Using the National Drug Code (NDC) number is a guaranteed way to ensure the right drug is pulled and used to fill the order. In addition, a bar code system is also common in today's practice and provides another safety feature.

MEDICATION SAFETY CONSIDERATION

When choosing a medication, either from a shelf or in an automated machine, using a check system of the NDC number between the printed label and the chosen bulk medication is the only way to verify the drug entered into the database and charged for is the same drug being used.

In addition to entering new drugs into the system, adjustments and changes will require data entry. There may be a need to increase or decrease a set reorder quantity for seasonal medications such as Tamiflu (for influenza) or Allegra (for allergies). In addition, there may be times when you are asked to identify a drug on the basis of a visual description. The database includes an **Image** feature that can be used to verify a medication.

■ Lab Objectives

In this Lab, you will:

- Demonstrate the process of adding a new drug into the database by its NDC number.
- Visually identify a drug by using the database *Image* feature.
- Explain common functions in inventory control including adjusting the ordered quantities of a drug, verifying the NDC and bar code numbers, and entering the product route of administration and dosage form.

ASHP goals: 11, 17, 26, 32, 33, 41, and 45.

■ Scenario

Today, you are working as the inventory technician, and several tasks need to be completed including some adjustments to reorders, new medications received in an order that must be entered into the database, and verification of medications that a patient has brought in.

■ Pre Lab Information

Read over the Lab completely, and identify and pull the drugs with which you will be working by their NDC numbers.

■ Student Directions

Estimated completion time: 30 minutes

1. Read through the steps in the Lab before performing the Lab exercise.
2. After reading through the Lab, perform the required steps to enter the new drug into the database.
3. Complete the exercise at the end of the Lab.

STEPS TO ADD A DRUG TO THE DATABASE

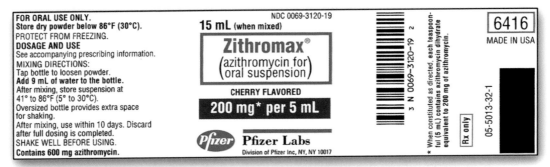

From Fulcher RM, Fulcher EM: *Math calculations for pharmacy technicians: a worktext*, 2 ed, St Louis, 2013, Saunders.

Use the above drug label to complete the following steps:

1. Access the main screen of Visual SuperScript.

2. Click on the **Drug** button located on the left side of the screen. A dialog box appears entitled *Drugs*. The *Drugs* form is used to maintain a database of drugs that are dispensed in the pharmacy.

3. Click on **Add Drug by NDC** located at the top left side of the form. A dialog box entitled *Add Drug by NDC* appears.

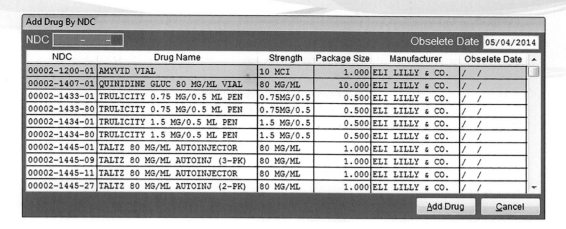

4. Enter the NDC number as it appears on the stock bottle label.

> Type *00069-3120-19* for azithromycin (Zithromax) 200 mg/5 mL oral suspension 15 mL.

5. Select the appropriate entry by clicking on the correct NDC number.

6. Click on **ADD DRUG** located at the bottom of the dialog box.

7. Click on the **EDIT** 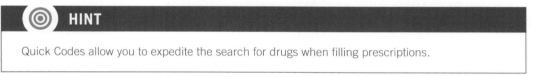 icon located at the top of the *Drugs* dialog box.

8. Tab to the *Quick Code* data entry field. Enter the first few characters of the drug name in the *Quick Code* data entry field.

> Enter *ZITOS* for azithromycin (Zithromax) oral suspension

◎ **HINT**

Quick Codes allow you to expedite the search for drugs when filling prescriptions.

Note: The *Alchemy Product ID* data entry field is automatically completed with the selection of the drug if an identification (ID) number has been assigned to the drug. In the practice setting, completing the entry in this field is important because this code produces all warning and counseling messages for the drug. Many other data entry fields are also automatically completed with the selection of the drug. The *Drug Class, Item Type, Gender,* and *Brand/Generic* data entry fields have been updated to coincide with the drug selection.

9. Tab to the *Default Sig* data entry field.

> Enter the abbreviation *T2TSP q12h* for *Take 2 teaspoons every 12 hours.*

Note: Certain drugs are frequently prescribed with the same instructions for use. Entering the appropriate instructions in the *Default Sig* data entry field can save time when filling a prescription.

10. Tab to the *Max Dose* (maximum dose) data entry field. Enter the maximum daily dose advised for this particular medication.

> Enter *500* for 500 mg.

11. Tab to the *Default Quantity* data entry field. Certain drugs are frequently prescribed with the same quantity instructions. Enter the desired quantity to be dispensed in the prescription for this particular medication.

> Enter *15* for the 15 mL container size as the default quantity for azithromycin (Zithromax) oral suspension

12. Tab to the *Default Day Supply* data entry field, and enter the desired quantity.

Enter 5.

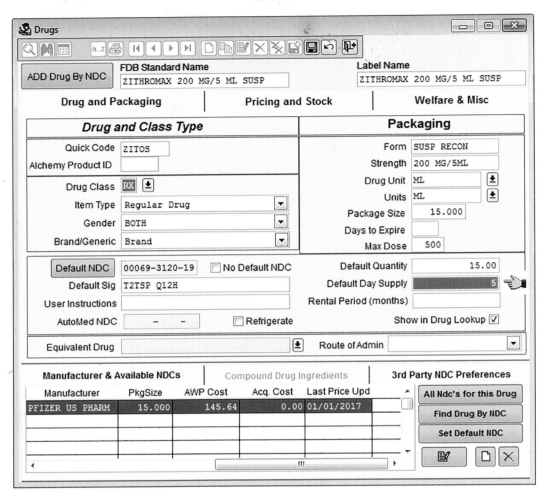

13. Click the **Pricing and Stock** tab located at the top of the form.

Note: The *Price Table* is a required data entry field that links each drug to a pricing formula for the purpose of calculating the usual and customary price of the drug. The correct *Price Table* has automatically been added with the selection of the drug.

14. In the **Track Inventory** tab, enter the *Minimum Stock* value that the pharmacy wishes to maintain for the new medication that is being added to the database.

Enter 5 in the *Regular Stock* column.

15. In the *Reorder Qty.* (reorder quantity) data entry field, enter the quantity of the medication that the pharmacy will reorder when the stock is at its minimum.

Enter 2 in the *Regular Stock* column.

16. Type the actual amount or quantity of medication that will be added to the pharmacy shelf in the *Last Verified Stock* data entry field.

> **Four stock bottles of azithromycin (Zithromax) will be added to the pharmacy shelf.**
>
> **Each bottle contains 15 mL.**
>
> **Therefore enter *60* for 60 mL in the *Last Verified Stock* data entry field.**

Note: The *Last Verified Stock* field is the amount of drug that is being added to the pharmacy shelf. This amount could be tablets, capsules, or liquid form (in milliliters).

Note: The tab **Welfare & Misc** located at the top of the form is not used for all drugs. This tab will be used when working with controlled substances and special considerations for Medicaid.

17. In the *Verification Date* data entry field, enter today's date and the time of day.

18. Click on the **Save** 💾 icon located at the top of the *Drugs* form. The new drug has now been added to the pharmacy's working drug file.

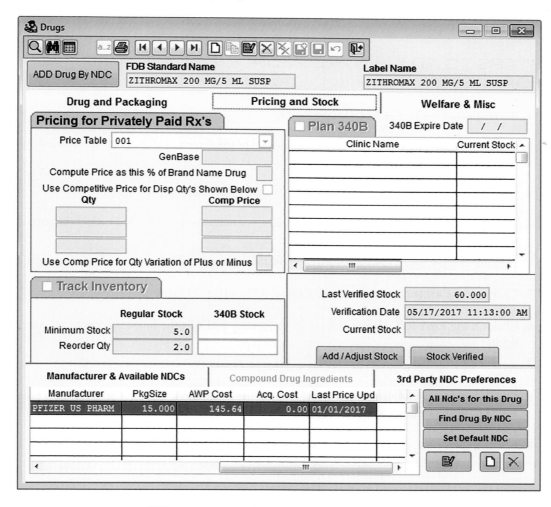

19. Click on the **Close** 🔌 icon located at the top of the *Drugs* form.

EXERCISE

Using the invoice for an order received in the pharmacy (see Lab 44 for the invoice), add the new drug *Fluocinonide 0.6% 30 g cream* to the pharmacy inventory. Appropriately apply stickers on the bottles. Adjust the quantities in stock for the other medications received to your pharmacy inventory. On completion of this exercise, submit the screenshots, stock bottles, and invoice for verification.

QUICK CHALLENGE

1. You have learned how to add drugs to the software database. In reading the steps in this Lab, you have come to understand that the pharmacy will order and update stock on a regular basis. Can you complete an electronic purchase order for ordering medication stock for the pharmacy?

2. Order the following stock from XYZ Drugs, Inc. Print the purchase order, and submit for verification.
   - Reorder Quantity: 56 Prempro 0.625/2.5 mg tab #00046-0875-6
   - Reorder Quantity: 200 Synthroid 137 mcg #00074-3727-19
   - Reorder Quantity: 90 Nexium 20 mg capsule #00186-5020-31

STEPS TO ADJUST THE REORDER QUANTITIES FOR A DRUG

1. Access the main screen of Visual SuperScript.

2. Click on the **DRUG** button located on the left side of the screen. A dialog box appears entitled *Drugs*.

3. Click on the **FIND** 🔍 icon at the top left of the *Drugs* dialog box.

4. Type the first three letters of the drug to search the database, and click **OK** to select the correct drug and dosage.

   Type *Zit* for Zithromax 250 mg z-pak tablet.

5. Click on the **PRICING AND STOCK** tab located at the top of the form.

6. Click on the **EDIT** 📝 icon at the top of the screen, and edit the following stock data entry fields:

   Change the amount in *Minimum Stock* to *24* and the *Reorder Qty.* to *48*.

7. Click on the **SAVE** 💾 icon located at the top of the *Drugs* form. The new drug has now been added to the pharmacy's working drug file.

8. Click on the **CLOSE** 🔼 icon located at the top of the *Drugs* form.

STEPS TO VERIFY DRUG IDENTITY

You have learned how to add new drugs to the software database, as well as change the order amount. In practice, a visual identification of a drug is required at times.

1. Access the main screen of Visual SuperScript.

2. Click on the **DRUG** button located on the left side of the screen. A dialog box appears entitled *Drugs*.

3. Click on the **FIND** 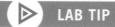 icon at the top left of the *Drugs* dialog box.

4. Type the first three letters of the drug to search the database, and click **OK** to select the correct drug and dosage.

Type *Lex* for Lexapro 20 mg tablets.

5. On the bottom right hand side of the screen, click on the **EDIT** icon. A box called *Drug NDC* appears that gives a general description of the medication.

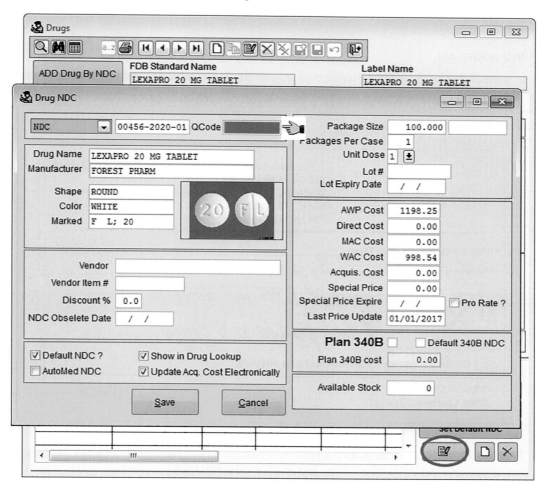

> ## ▷ LAB TIP
>
> The **EDIT** button that is used for a drug image is at the bottom of the screen and is not the one at the top of the *Drugs* box.

EXERCISE

Mrs. Brown is an older patient who lives alone and often brings her "brown bag" of medications to the pharmacy for identification. Use the **DRUG IMAGE** tab and the following profile list of her medications to give her a description of each medication.

- Prevacid, 30 mg capsule DR
- Tegretol, 200 mg tablets
- Risperdal, 2 mg tablets
- Neurontin, 300 mg capsule

Print a screen shot of the *Drug NDC* dialog box for each drug for this assignment.

LAB 6

Entering and Preparing New Prescriptions in a Community Setting

▪ Introduction

The community pharmacy setting is designed around dispensing **prescriptions** that are handwritten or electronically written and sent to a pharmacy by a physician. The prescription, or RX, must contain certain information by law and is specific for a patient. Some of the major components of a prescription are the following:

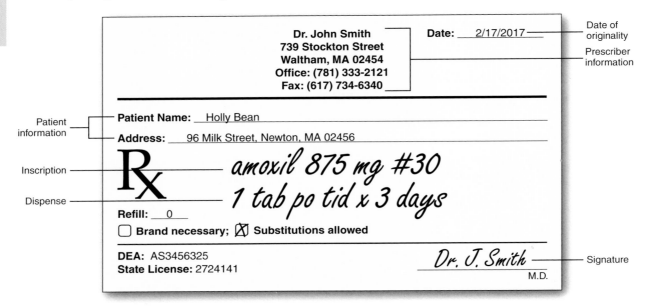

- **Prescriber information:** Includes the prescriber address, phone number, and Drug Enforcement Administration (DEA) number. (Refer to Lab 2 for the verification process.)
- **Patient information:** Includes the patient's name and address.
- **Date of originality:** Prescriptions normally expire 1 year from the date of origin, and prescriptions for some controlled substances must be filled or refilled within 6 months.
- **Brand necessary:** The physician must handwrite or choose "Brand necessary" if he or she specifically chooses this medication.

MEDICATION SAFETY CONSIDERATION

If a patient brings in a prescription, but it was written a significant time before the date he or she is requesting its first fill, then ask the following questions: "Why have you saved this prescription for months before filling it?" "Do you still need the prescription filled?" Check to see whether the patient has refills on file in the patient profile.

- **Superscription:** The symbol RX means, "Take this."
- **Inscription:** Includes the medication name, strength, dosage form, and how much is needed or how many days to supply.
- **Subscription:** Includes directions if the medication needs special preparation such as a compounded ointment or cream.

- **Sig** or **Signa-:** Refers to a special language or code that requires interpretation and is similar to a shorthand that must be transcribed. For example "Take 1 po bid" means "Take 1 tablet by mouth twice daily."
- **Signature:** The prescription must have the actual signature of the prescriber (physician, dentist, physician assistant [PA], or nurse assistant).

■ Lab Objectives

In this Lab, you will:

- Demonstrate how to perform necessary computer functions to enter a new prescription into a pharmacy system.
- Learn shortcuts to be used when entering **SIGS**.
- Apply rules for noncontrolled and controlled medications when filling and preparing for dispensing.
- Demonstrate the technician's role in the medication use process.
- Correctly interpret and calculate prescriptions for preparation.
- Apply billing techniques to written prescriptions when performing data entry (e.g., third party, cash, Medicare/Medicaid).

■ Scenario

Today, you are working in a busy retail pharmacy and will receive several prescriptions that will need to be prepared for patient pick up. Using the knowledge you have gained and the data skills you have performed to date, you will enter each one into the patient's profile, create a label, and then prepare the medication by counting or pouring.

 LAB TIP

Using the shortcut abbreviations made for the software will save time, which is very important in a busy store. See the Sig Abbreviations chart in the front of the book for the chart once you have interpreted the prescription but before the entry process begins. Example: typing simply "AP1-2GD" would be the same as typing "Apply 1 or 2 drops daily."

■ Pre Lab Information

Regardless of the practice setting for the pharmacy technician and pharmacist, entering data into the computer is a major component of their workloads. In the retail setting, for example, a customer drops off the prescription hard copy. After the pharmacy technician has obtained all of the necessary information from the customer, information is entered into the computer. This Lab explains the steps involved in filling new prescriptions.

Working through the steps involved in interpreting and transcribing a prescription is beneficial before completing this Lab.

■ Student Directions

Estimated completion time: 1.5 hour

1. Read through the steps in the Lab before performing the Lab exercise.
2. Using the Sig Abbreviations chart in the front of the book for abbreviations or codes, interpret the prescription directions, and decide what should be typed out in the **SIG IN ENGLISH** data entry field.
3. Perform the required steps to create a label, and prepare the product for dispensing.
4. Enter and prepare the additional prescriptions provided at the end of the Lab.

Dr. John Thompson
81 Highland Street
Allston, MA 02134
Office: (617) 632-4568
Fax: (617) 734-6340

Date: _2/17/2017_

Patient Name: _Kenneth Sharpe_

Address: _888 James Street, Allston, MA_

R͟x   *Lipitor 40 mg, 1 hs #30*
       Brand necessary

Refill: _2_

DEA: AT4278431
State License: 3445542

Dr. J. Thompson
M.D.

Use the above prescription to complete the following steps.

1. Access the main screen of Visual SuperScript.

2. Click on **FILL RX'S** located on the left side of the menu screen. The *Select Available Pharmacist* box appears. Click on the arrow, and choose any available pharmacist. Click **OK**. The *Prescription Processing* form appears.

3. Click on the **NEW RX** 🗋 icon on the top left of the *Prescription Processing* form.

   Note: Prescription information such as the **RX NO.** (prescription number) and **DISPENSE DATE** are automatically generated and added to the form. Tab to the **RX ORIGIN** data entry field from the drop-down menu. In this case, the prescription is *Written*.

4. Tab to the next data field. This is the **CUSTOMER LOOKUP** text box. Type the first three letters of the customer's last name, and hit **ENTER**.

   Type *SHA* for Kenneth Sharpe as indicated in the sample prescription.

5. Select the appropriate customer by clicking on the customer name or by clicking **OK** when the customer name is highlighted in blue.

   Note: The customer's personal information such as **ADDRESS**, **PHONE**, and **BIRTHDATE** will be automatically added to the *Prescription Processing* form.

   Note: You are automatically directed to the **DOCTOR** text box once the patient information is populated. For new prescriptions, the system will search the patient's prescription file to find the name of the prescriber of the most recently filled prescription. If found, then the system will insert the prescriber's name into this field. If a different physician has written the new prescription, then you can delete the old name and enter the new one. For this particular exercise, enter the physician, Dr. John Thompson, who is listed in the sample prescription.

6. Press the **TAB** key. You will be prompted to the **PRESCRIBED DRUG** data entry field. Type the first three letters of the prescribed drug into the **PRESCRIBED DRUG** data entry field. Then press **ENTER**.

   Enter *Lip* for Kenneth Sharpe's Lipitor.

7. Select the appropriate drug from the *Drug Name Lookup* dialog box by double-clicking on the drug name or selecting the drug name and clicking **OK**. Remember, the physician specified "Brand necessary"; consequently, when the drop-down menu offers the choices, choose the brand name, Lipitor, not the generic drug name, atorvastatin.

 LAB TIP

If a series of warning dialog boxes appear, these are known as drug utilization reviews (DURs). The patient's medication history is compared against the drug you are entering for pregnancy warnings, drug-drug and drug-food interactions, or contraindication conditions or diseases. (The warning messages should be viewed and approved by the pharmacist before dispensing the medication.)

8. After receiving approval from the instructor (simulated pharmacist review) to continue, click on close to move through the warnings.

9. Brand and generic drugs will appear under *Available Drug Choices*. Use your keyboard's up and down keys to highlight the drug option you want. Press **ENTER**, and the full drug information will appear below, along with an image if available. Choose the generic substitution unless the physician has specified—dispense as written (DAW).

 HINT

Ensure that the price feeds in the drug information. If it does not, click on the **RECALC** button to populate the *Price* field. Otherwise, you may get an error when you transmit the prescription.

10. Next, you will be prompted to the **REFILLS ORDERED** data entry field.

   Key in the appropriate number of refills.

11. Press the **TAB** key. You will be prompted to enter the **PRESCRIBED QUANTITY**.

   Key in the appropriate quantity in the **PRESCRIBED QUANTITY** data entry field.

12. In the **DAW** text box, choose the correct **DAW** code by clicking on the arrow on the right side of the **DAW** data entry field.

   Click on the correct DAW code from the drop-down menu.

Note: When filling a prescription, knowing the correct **DAW** code to be assigned to a prescription is necessary for reimbursement. To accomplish this, distinguish between the brand name and the generic name of the medication. Although the prescriber may write the brand name of a drug on a patient's prescription, it may not necessarily mean that the brand-name drug must be dispensed. If the prescriber indicates **DAW** or "brand name medically necessary" on the patient's prescription for a brand-name drug, then the brand-name drug rather than the generic alternative MUST be dispensed. **This situation, for example, would be a DAW code 1.** Failure to use the proper **DAW** code may result in improper third-party reimbursement to the pharmacy. Seven **DAW** codes are used in the pharmacy practice:

DAW 0—Prescriber has approved the dispensing of a generic medication.

DAW 1—Prescriber requests that the brand-name drug be dispensed.

DAW 2—Prescriber has approved the dispensing of a generic drug, but the patient has requested that the brand-name drug be dispensed.

DAW 3—Pharmacist dispenses the drug as written.

DAW 4—No generic drugs are available in the store.

DAW 5—Brand-name drug is dispensed but is priced as a generic drug.

DAW 6—Registered pharmacist (RPh)–prescriber call is attempted.

13. Press the **TAB** key. Type the patient abbreviated directions in the **SIG** text box.

> *Key in T1T PO HS as the shortcut abbreviation* SIG *for Kenneth Sharpe.*

Note: What appears in the blue **SIG IN ENGLISH** space is what will appear on the label. If an error is made when typing in the **SIG**, then backspace to delete the error and retype the correct information.

14. Press the **TAB** key. You will be prompted to enter **PRESCRIBED DAYS SUPPLY**. Type in the appropriate days' supply in the **PRESCRIBED DAYS SUPPLY** data entry field.

> *Enter 30 for Kenneth Sharpe's* PRESCRIBED DAYS SUPPLY.

 LAB TIP

Days' supply involves calculating the number of days that a particular prescription will last. All third-party payers require this information. Failure to provide the prescribed days' supply information properly may result in the pharmacy losing money. To calculate the days' supply that a prescription will last, use the following formula:

$$\text{Days' supply} = \frac{\text{Total quantity dispensed}}{\text{Total quantity taken per day}}$$

The days' supply is the number of days a medication will last for one filling. Days' supply does not take into account refills. The majority of the third-party payers will reimburse a pharmacy for a 30-day supply of a medication.

Note: In the **RX NOTES** section, you may add any notes that apply. Most states require patients to receive the opportunity for medication counseling. The **RX NOTES** section is a good place to document "offered counseling, but patient refused counseling" or other similar important information.

15. Press the **ENTER** key. Click the **SAVE** 💾 icon.

 HINT

Make sure you save using the **SAVE** button to the right. (Save this prescription in the system memory.) The **SAVE** button on the left will save the entry and automatically move you to a new prescription for the same customer. If you use the **SAVE** button on the left and the screen goes blank, then you can click the **BACK** button to reclaim the prescription and print the label.

16. Before recording the prescription, take note of the prescription number. You will need this number to print the label. Click on the **XMIT/RECORD** on the left of the screen to complete adjudication. The screen will clear and prepare to fill a new prescription. Click **LABEL/PRINT**, enter the prescription number noted previously, and print the label after verifying the information.

17. Prepare the medication for dispensing, including labeling the product. Affix the second label to the back of the original prescription.

EXERCISE

Enter the prescriptions and prepare the products for dispensing using the following assigned prescriptions. Leave the stock bottle, original prescription, and prepared product for a final check by the pharmacist. Remember to affix the second label on the back of the original prescription in your book.

Practice using the abbreviation shortcuts found in the Sig Abbreviations chart in the front of the book to make the process quicker. All drug community software programs use these abbreviations to save time. Some prescriptions may require adding new patient information, new prescriber information, or adding a new drug to the database. You may review previous Labs for these procedures.

Dr. Jasmine Abbosh
836 Farmington Avenue
Worcester, MA 01601
Office: (617) 232-9911
Fax: (617) 734-6340

Date: ___2/17/2017___

Patient Name: ___Richard Clemens___

Address: ___345 Fenwick Dr, Chestnut Hill, MA 02167___

Rx

Zithromax 250 mg 2 tabs po now, then 1 tab po qd x 4 days
Brand necessary

Refill: ___0___

DEA: BA4884533

Dr. J. Abbosh
M.D.

Dr. Kareem Babu
300 Stainford Street
Springfield, MA 01104
Office: (413) 776-9000
Fax: (413) 776-9001

Date: ___2/17/2017___

Patient Name: ___Larry Jones___

Address: ___63 Birch Street, Wellesley, MA 02482___

Rx

Bactroban 2% ung
22 g tube AAA bid ud

Refill: ___0___

DEA: BB5723469
State License: 2724141

Dr. K. Babu
M.D.

Dr. Antoine Diallo
5500 Maryland Street
Bethesda, MA 20814
Office: (301) 725-3458
Fax: (301) 725-3458

Date: _2/17/2017_

Patient Name: _Miguel Sanchez_

Address: _75 Tremont Street, Cambridge, MA 02139_

℞ *Humulin R inject 15 units*
sq tid ac (Spanish label required)

Refill: _3_

DEA: AD1234567

Dr. A. Diallo
M.D.

Dr. Stephen Hardy
76 Walnut Street
Allston, MA 02134
Office: (617) 532-6390
Fax: (617) 734-6340

Date: _2/17/2017_

Patient Name: _Margaret Noonan_

Address: _30 Inman Street, Brighton, MA 02135_

℞ *etanercept 25 mg kit #1 ud*

Refill: _0_

DEA: AH4442149RES
State License: 4525253

Dr. S. Hardy
M.D.

Dr. Robert Cornish
1789 Hyde Avenue
Allston, MA 02134
Office: (617) 372-7650
Fax: (617) 734-6340

Date: 2/17/2017

Patient Name: Bernice Good

Address: 92 Fernwood Terrace, Allston, MA 02134

Rx

blood glucose meter, lancets, strips

Refill: 0 ud

DEA: ACS5433230
State License: 7665899

Dr. R. Cornish
M.D.

Dr. Karen Davis
132 Hines Street
Newton, MA 02456
Office: (617) 553-4300
Fax: (617) 734-6340

Date: 2/17/2017

Patient Name: Verna Bushey

Address: 68 Birch Street, Newton, MA 02456

Rx

Compazine 25 mg supp #XII
1 pr bid for n/v

Refill: 0

DEA: AD4252261
State License: 3562215

Dr. K. Davis
M.D.

LAB 7

Processing a New Prescription for a Patient with a Third-Party Payment Type

■ Introduction

In the community practice setting, processing a third-party claim for a prescription can be a challenging part of the daily tasks. Communicating with the patient and third-party company will be necessary for additional information, claim rejections, and formulary concerns with many of the prescriptions being filled. Customers will need to provide their card for verification or call the company to talk directly with the physician's office or insurance provider.

Processing payments with insurance companies, which includes inputting the most current and correct information possible for both the patient and the third-party provider, is one of the pharmacy technician's common daily tasks, as well as asking questions and receiving answers when needed. Assisting the pharmacist in this area is key to a good workflow and can prevent errors.

MEDICATION SAFETY CONSIDERATION

Always check the National Drug Code (NDC) number for the prescription you are filling, (counting or pouring); the NDC number is the KEY identifier for processing an insurance payment.

■ Lab Objectives

In this Lab, you will:

- Demonstrate the process of filling a prescription and of entering data for a patient with a third-party payment type.
- Learn how to identify necessary information from a sample insurance card, and discuss how to interpret and manage a rejection (e.g., codes).
- Discuss what a formulary is and the common types of medications found within.

■ Pre Lab Information

Entering and verifying third-party or insurance data when processing a prescription is a major component of the community or retail setting. For instance, when a customer drops off the prescription hard copy, the customer will present a card containing pertinent information if he or she has an insurance plan that covers the cost of the prescription. This plan may be a third-party company through an employer, Medicaid from the state, or Medicare Part D.

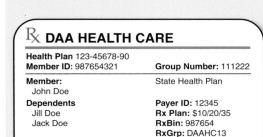

 LAB TIP

Refer to Lab 4 for more third-party card samples. You will need to identify the KEY information required to enter into the patient's profile.

After the pharmacy technician has obtained or verified all the necessary information from the customer, such as *member identification (ID) number*, *group number*, *copay requirements*, and *coverage information*, the prescription data are entered into the computer.

 LAB TIP

This Lab explains the steps involved in filling a new prescription for a customer with insurance. Working through the steps involved in interpreting and transcribing a prescription (see Lab 6) before completing the following Lab is beneficial.

■ **Student Directions**

Estimated completion time: 30 minutes

1. Read through the steps in the Lab before performing the Lab exercise.
2. After reading through the Lab, perform the required steps to create a label and to prepare the product for dispensing.
3. Complete the exercise at the end of the Lab.

Dr. John Thompson
81 Highland Street
Allston, MA 02134
Office: (617) 632-4568
Fax: (617) 734-6340

Date: ___2/17/2017___

Patient Name: ___Brian Davidson___

Address: ___27 Bradford Street, Newton, MA___

R̶x *Ceftin 500 mg, qd #30*
      Brand necessary

Refill: ___0___

DEA: AT4278431
State License: 3445542

Dr. J. Thompson
M.D.

Use the above prescription to complete the following steps.

1. Access the main screen of Visual SuperScript.

2. Click on **FILL RX'S** located on the left side of the menu screen. The *Prescription Processing* form appears.

3. Select the appropriate pharmacist on call. In this case, choose *CAROL* from the drop-down menu. Click **OK**. This will launch the *Prescription Processing* form.

4. Click on the **NEW RX** 🗋 icon on the top left of the *Prescription Processing* form.

   Note: Prescription information such as the **Rx No.** (prescription number) and **DISPENSE DATE** are automatically generated and added to the form.

5. Ensure that your initials appear in the *Tech/Rph Init* data entry field that appears, and click **OK**. You may also choose the **RX ORIGIN** (DROPCAP) from the drop-down menu if the prescription is not written.

6. Tab to the next data field. This is the **CUSTOMER LOOKUP** text box. Type the first three letters of the customer's last name, and hit **ENTER**.

   Type *DAV* for Brian Davidson as indicated in the sample prescription.

7. Select the appropriate customer by double-clicking on the customer name or by clicking **OK** when the customer name is highlighted in blue.

   Note: The customer's personal information such as **ADDRESS**, **PHONE**, and **BIRTHDATE** will be automatically added to the *Prescription Processing* form.

   Note: You are automatically directed to the **DOCTOR** text box once the patient information is populated. For new prescriptions, the system will search the patient's prescription file to find the name of the prescriber of the most recently filled prescription. If found, then the system will insert the prescriber's name into this field. If a different physician has written the new prescription, then you can delete the old name and enter the new one.

8. Search for *Thompson, John* in the **Doctor** text box as indicated on the prescription on the previous page.

9. Press the **Tab** key. You will be prompted to the **Prescribed Drug** data entry field. Type the first three letters of the prescribed drug into the **Prescribed Drug** data entry field. Then press **Enter**.

   Enter *Cef* for Brian's Cefaclor.

10. Select the appropriate drug from the *Drug Name Lookup* dialog box by double-clicking on the drug name or by selecting the drug name and clicking **OK**.

 LAB TIP

If a series of warning dialog boxes appear, then these are known as drug utilization reviews (DURs). The patient's medication history is compared against the drug you are entering for pregnancy warnings, drug-drug and drug-food interactions, or contraindication conditions or diseases. (The warning messages should be viewed and approved by the pharmacist before dispensing the medication.)

11. After receiving approval from the instructor to continue, click **Close** to move through the warnings.

12. The drug name will appear under **Available Drug Choices**. Press **Enter** and full drug information appears below, along with an image if available. Choose the generic substitution unless the physician has specified dispense as written (DAW).

13. Next, you will be prompted to the **Refills Ordered** data entry field.

   Key in the appropriate number of refills.

14. Press the **Tab** key. You will be prompted to enter the **Prescribed Quantity**.

   Key in the appropriate quantity in the Prescribed Quantity data entry field.

15. In the **DAW** text box, choose the correct **DAW** code by clicking on the arrow on the right side of the **DAW** data entry field.

   Click on the correct DAW code from the drop-down menu.

Note: When filling a prescription, knowing the correct **DAW** code to be assigned to a prescription is necessary for reimbursement. To accomplish this, distinguish between the brand name and the generic name of the medication. Although the prescriber may write the brand name of a drug on a patient's prescription, it may not necessarily mean that the brand-name drug must be dispensed. If the prescriber indicates **DAW** or "brand name medically necessary" on the patient's prescription for a brand-name drug, then the brand-name drug rather than the generic alternative MUST be dispensed. This situation, for example, would be a **DAW** code 1. Failure to use the proper **DAW** code may result in improper third-party reimbursement to the pharmacy. Seven **DAW** codes are used in the pharmacy practice:

DAW 0—Prescriber has approved the dispensing of a generic medication.

DAW 1—Prescriber requests that the brand-name drug be dispensed.

DAW 2—Prescriber has approved the dispensing of a generic drug, but the patient has requested that the brand-name drug be dispensed.

DAW 3—Pharmacist dispenses the drug as written.

DAW 4—No generic drugs are available in the store.

DAW 5—Brand-name drug is dispensed but is priced as a generic drug.

DAW 6—Registered pharmacist (RPh)–prescriber call is attempted.

16. Type the patient abbreviated directions in the **Sig** text box.

Key in **T1T QD PO** *as the shortcut abbreviation* S_IG_ *for Brian Davidson.*

Note: What appears in the blue **Sig in English** space is what will appear on the label. If an error is made when typing in the **Sig**, then backspace to delete the error and retype the correct information.

17. Press the **Tab** key. You will be prompted to enter **Prescribed Days Supply**. Type in the appropriate days' supply in the **Prescribed Days Supply** data entry field.

Enter **30** *for Brian Davidson's* P_RESCRIBED_ D_AYS_ S_UPPLY_.

 LAB TIP

Days' supply involves calculating the number of days that a particular prescription will last. All third-party payers require this information. Failure to provide the prescribed days' supply information properly may result in the pharmacy losing money. To calculate the days' supply that a prescription will last, use the following formula:

$$\text{Days' supply} = \frac{\text{Total quantity dispensed}}{\text{Total quantity taken per day}}$$

The days' supply is the number of days a medication will last for one filling. Days' supply does not take into account refills. The majority of the third-party payers will reimburse a pharmacy for a 30-day supply of a medication.

Note: In the **Rx Notes** section, you may add any notes that apply. Most states require patients to receive the opportunity for medication counseling. The **Rx Notes** section is a good place to document "offered counseling, but patient refused counseling" or other similar important information.

18. Press the **Enter** key. Click the **Save** 💾 icon.

 LAB TIP

The **Save** button on the left will save the entry and automatically move you to a new prescription for the same customer. If you use the **Save** button on the left and the screen goes blank, then you can click the **Back** button to reclaim the prescription and print the label. If you inadvertently hit the **Back** button, it will revert back to the last screen and prescription.

19. Before recording the prescription, take note of the prescription number. You will need this number to print the label. Click on the **Xmit/Record** button on the left of the screen to complete adjudication. The screen will clear and prepare to fill a new prescription. Click **Label/Print**, enter the prescription number previously noted, and print the label after verifying the information.

20. Prepare the medication for dispensing, including labeling the product. Affix the second label to the back of the original prescription.

Note: The label has two amounts: (1) price and (2) copay. These reflect the amount the insurance allows for the drug (price) and the amount the customer must pay as his or her part (copay).

EXERCISE

Scenario 1: Refill too soon.

A patient is requesting a refill too soon on insurance, and the Pharmacist must override this restriction if he believes it is appropriate. The patient states she lost her medication that was filled last week. Since this is a maintenance medication for heart disease, he instructs you to process the prescription.

1. First, to simulate this rejection, fill the following prescription on her insurance using directions found in this lab.

2. Change the prescription date to a week ago, and the dispense date to 2 weeks ago.

Agner, Millie, Amitriptyline HCL 10 mg tablet one hs #30, 2 refills
Dr. Crusoe, Jonathan

3. Do not forget to process the prescription through the insurance by choosing the **Xmit/Record** tab after saving the record.

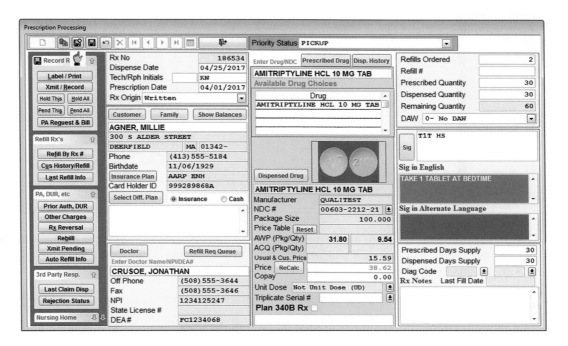

4. From the left-hand side, choose the **Cus History/Refill** button. Using the patient's name to pull history, look up the Amitriptyline Rx and click the check box to the left of the Rx #.

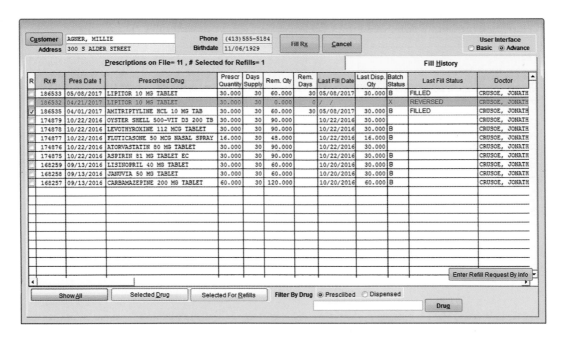

5. Since she is asking for another refill, click **Fill Rx** after marking it.

6. The message, **WARNING! Refill Too Soon**, appears.

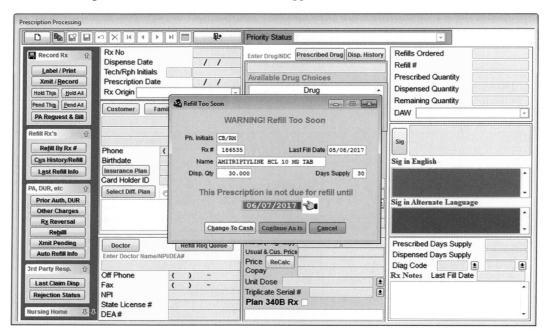

7. The Pharmacist has agreed to fill the prescription and instructs you to process the refill. Click **Continue As Is**, and then click on **Xmit/Record**. The following screen appears. Click the red **X** in the upper right-hand corner or the **Close** button.

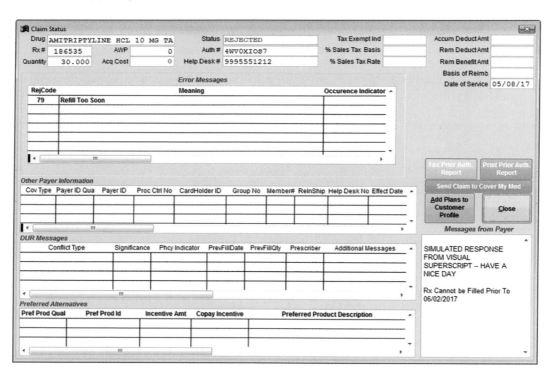

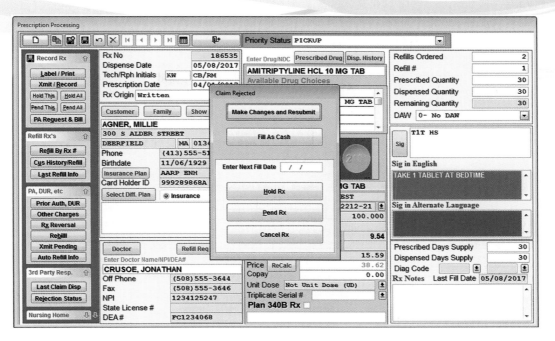

8. Click on **Make Changes and Resubmit**. You are returned to the *Prescription Processing* dialog box. Click the **Prior Auth, DUR** button on the left side of the screen.

To override and allow the refill, a prior authorization code must be input. The Registered Pharmacist (RPh) can override the restriction by placing code 04 in place of the 01 under **Submission Clarification Codes**. Close the *Priority Authorization, DUR, etc* dialog box by clicking on the red **X** in the upper right-hand corner.

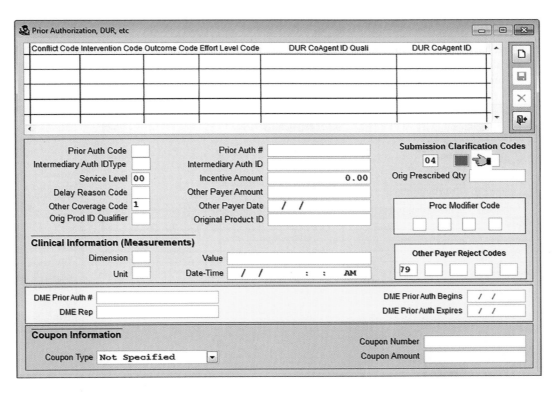

9. Click on **Xmit/Record** again. The following screen appears. The prescription is now **Paid**; the prescription label can now be printed.

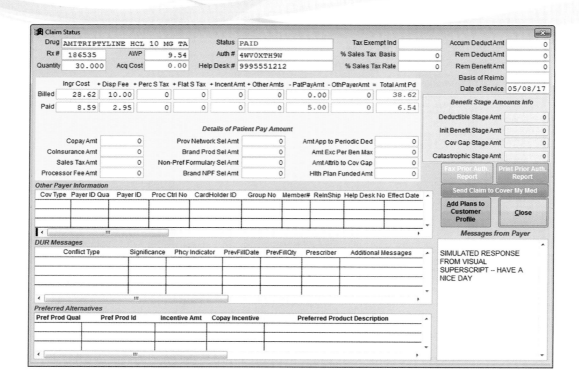

Scenario 2: Drug Utilization Reviews and Third-Party Rejection for Drug-Pregnancy Alert

Dr. Nobel Lasalle has telephoned in two new prescriptions for Tanya Bramwell:

Coumadin 2.5 mg, 1 qd #30, specifying "Brand necessary" with two refills

Doxepin 25 mg, 1 hs #30, specifying "Brand necessary" with two refills

Note: Save the first prescription with the left-side **SAVE** button that contains the plus sign. This will allow you to add a second prescription with prefilled information for the patient and doctor. Record each prescription number.

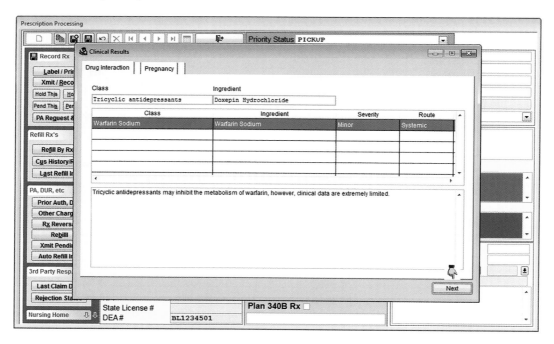

The *Clinical Results* dialog box appears with a warning message. The drug utilization review (DUR) warning is a therapeutic duplication for the doxepin in her history. The Pharmacist must review and decide whether the two medications can be taken together or to call the physician to change or discuss.

The *Clinical Results* dialog box actually contains two warnings on two different tabs: (1) Drug Interaction and (2) Pregnancy. The next warning is **Serious Pregnancy Warning Found** because she is a female patient between 18 and 45 years of age.

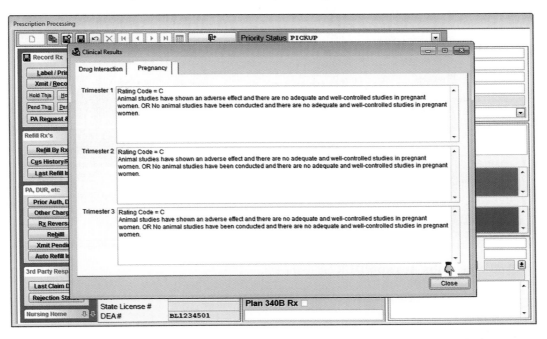

Community Pharmacy Practice

Pharmacist instructs you to continue with the prescription after a discussion with the patient. Click the right-sided **Save** button. Remember to note the prescription numbers before closing. Click the **Xmit/Record** button to process the prescription through her insurance. It is rejected, displaying code 88, which means "DUR Reject Error" for a Drug-Pregnancy Alert.

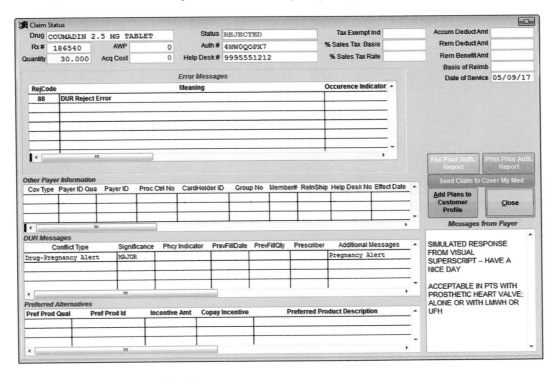

Close the *Claim Status* dialog box.

The following screen will appear and will require you to click **MAKE CHANGES AND RESUBMIT**.

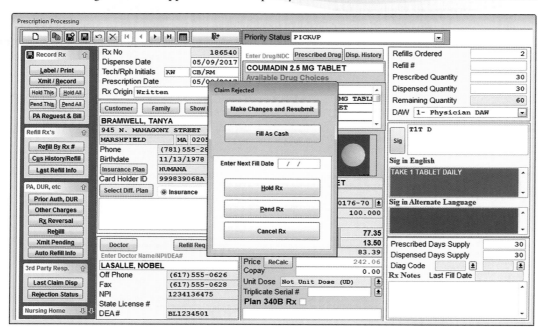

Choose the **PRIOR AUTHOR/DUR** tab to the left.

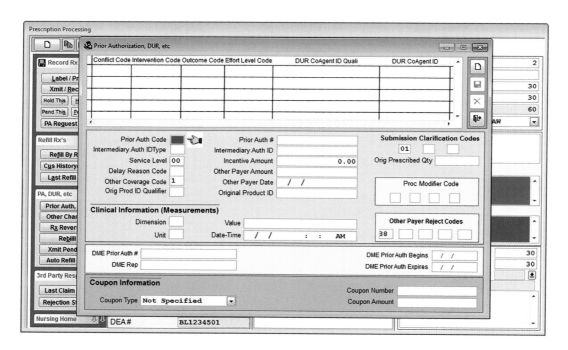

Community Pharmacy Practice

Click on the **New Rx** 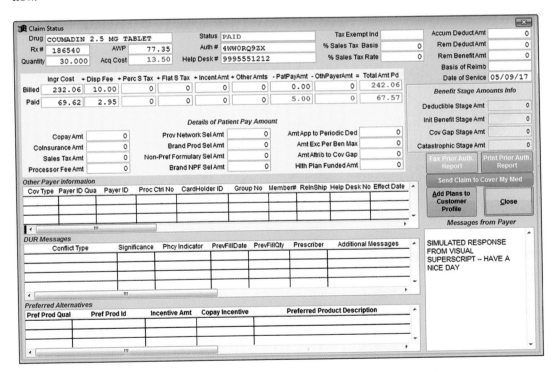 icon on the right-hand side of the screen. In the **Prior Authorization, DUR, etc** Table, enter the following conflict codes as shown below. Click the **Save** icon.

PG, M0, 1A

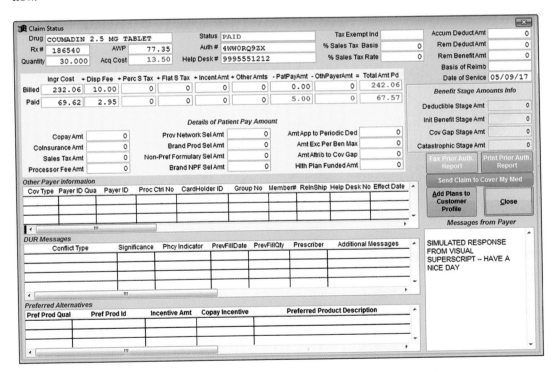

Close the **Prior Authorization, DUR, etc** screen, and click the **Xmit/Record** to process now.

The prescription is now **Paid**, and the prescription label can now be printed.

EXERCISE

Enter the prescriptions and prepare the products for dispensing using the following assigned prescriptions. Leave the stock bottle, original prescription, and prepared product for a final check by the pharmacist.

The customer's personal information such as **ADDRESS**, **PHONE**, and **BIRTHDATE** will automatically be added to the *Prescription Processing* form, but you will need to verify the insurance coverage by reviewing the card information and making any changes as required.

Note: Practice using the abbreviation shortcuts found in the Sig Abbreviations chart in the front of the book to make the process quicker. All drug community software programs use these abbreviations to save time. Some prescriptions may require adding new patient information, new prescriber information, or adding a new drug to the database. You may review previous Labs for these procedures.

▶ LAB TIP

Remember to affix the second label on the back of the original prescription as you verify the label against the bottle and the prescription one last time. Look at drug name, patient name, and date of birth (DOB), and drug NDC number. Have a fellow student check your work.

Dr. Jasmine Abbosh
836 Farmington Avenue
Worcester, MA.01601
860-232-9911
BA4892433

For: Floyd Ellis

Address: 73 Birch St. Worcester, MA.   Date: 3/21/17

Glucophage 500mg ÷ qd #30
Folic Acid ÷ mg #30
Inderal 40mg ÷ bid #60
Zyloprim 300mg ÷ qd #30

REFILL ___4___ TIMES   Dr. Jasmine Abbosh

M.D.

Dr. Robert Hendrickson
1324 Maynard Road
Waltham, MA. 02454
781-372-5311
AH5434547

For: Kevin Anderson

Address: 526 Maple St. Waltham, MA. Date: 5-4-17

Cialis 10mg
Sig: take ÷ prior to anticipated
sexual activity #30

REFILL __2__ TIMES   _Dr. Hendrickson_   M.D.

Dr. Jasmine Abbosh
836 Farmington Avenue
Worcester, MA.01601
860-232-9911
BA4892433

For: Maxine Broswell

Address: 75 Pinewood Terr Worcester Date: 4-6-17

Humira 40mg
Sig: inj subcutaneous g every other week

REFILL __8__ TIMES   _Dr. Jasmine Abbosh_   M.D.

Dr. Ramon Ramirez
134 Boylston Street
Cambridge, MA. 02139
617-479-3400
AR3587726

For: Michael Duke

Address: 123 Washington Street Cambridge *Date:* 3-3-17

℞   Ciproxen 200mg #10 x 1 week

REFILL ___0___ TIMES   Dr. R. Ramirez

                                      M.D.

Dr. Robert Hendrickson
1324 Maynard Road
Waltham, MA. 02454
781-372-5311
AH5434547

For: Gary Nardone

Address: 381 Freeman St. Waltham, MA. *Date:* 9-1-17

℞   Cephalexin   500mg
         Disp: #18
         Sig: 2 stat, then ÷ tid starting tomorrow

REFILL __x1__ TIMES   Dr. Robert Hendrick.

                                        M.D.

Dr. Ramon Ramirez
134 Boylston Street
Cambridge, MA. 02139
617-479-3400
AR3587726

For: Patricia Armstrong

Address: 23 Egmont St Cambridge, MA   Date: 5-22-17

Prozac 20mg #60
Sig: ÷ AM, ÷ NOON pc
DESYREL 50mg #30
Sig: ii or iii hs pc

REFILL _0_ TIMES   _____ M.D.

Dr. Stanton Yeager
295 Chestnut St.
Newton, MA. 02456
617-445-5566
AY7732262

For: Peter Allen

Address: 53 Walnut St. Newton, MA. 02456   Date: 5-1-17

Ceftin susp.
Sig: ÷ tsp q12 hrs. x7 days

REFILL _0_ TIMES   _Dr. Stan Yeager_ M.D.

LAB 8

Drug Utilization Review Using Electronic Patient Profiles

■ Introduction

Patient profiles are only as complete as you make them, and using the ability to add notes and over-the-counter (OTC) medications, vitamins, herbals, and durable and nondurable products, such as insulin needles or lancets, is the best practice for a complete patient history. All medications, including those not actually dispensed at your pharmacy, can be compared by the system for drug-drug interaction, allergies, drug-food interactions, and disease states. This process is known as a *drug utilization review* (DUR). As you learned in Lab 6, if any of these situations exists, then the database provides an alert at the bottom of the screen. Keeping a complete record, including notes such as demographic information, pregnancy status, and disease states, is necessary to provide the pharmacist with a complete picture of the patient and the conditions he or she may have. If a condition shows a contraindication with the drug being entered, then a DUR message will be revealed.

For example: *Patient profile in system:* Karen Anderson. Date of birth (DOB): 8.3.73.

She brings a new prescription in for amoxicillin (antibiotic), and her current profile lists her medications as Ortho-Evra (birth-control patch). A DUR comes up on the screen when trying to enter the amoxicillin because the profile indicates her age as appropriate for child-bearing age.

Because the woman is of child-bearing age, based on the profile information, the screen shows a DUR once the amoxicillin is entered in the drug field. In this case, the technician should immediately stop the prescription entry process and notify the pharmacist to decide whether this prescription could cause a problem if taken. If not, then the pharmacy will allow the prescription data entry process to continue. If the pharmacist speaks with the patient and determines child-bearing status as a possible contraindication, then the physician needs to be consulted.

Dr. Robert Hendrickson 1324 Maynard Road Waltham, MA 02454 Office: (781) 372-5311 Fax: (781) 372-5310	**Date:** ___2/17/2017___

Patient Name: ___Karen Anderson___

Address: ___526 Maple Street, Waltham, MA 02354___

℞   *amoxicillin 500 mg, 1 tid #21*

Refill: ___0___

DEA: AH434547
State License: 026577

Dr. R. Hendrickson
                M.D.

MEDICATION SAFETY CONSIDERATION

The U.S. Food and Drug Administration (FDA) has established five different categories to indicate whether a drug would harm a women or fetus. If the profile is complete, then each time a new drug is entered, the system will check the drug against any other existing drug for drug-drug interactions and also against the patient profile information such as age and sex,* which only works if the profile is complete.

CATEGORY A

Adequate and well-controlled studies have failed to demonstrate a risk to the fetus in the first trimester of pregnancy. (No evidence suggests a risk in later trimesters.)

CATEGORY B

Animal reproduction studies have failed to demonstrate a risk to the fetus, and no adequate and well-controlled studies in pregnant women have been conducted.

CATEGORY C

Animal reproduction studies have shown an adverse effect on the fetus. No adequate and well-controlled studies in humans have been conducted, but potential benefits may warrant the use of the drug in pregnant women, despite its potential risks.

CATEGORY D

Positive evidence of human fetal risk exists, based on adverse reaction data from investigational or marketing experience or studies in humans, but potential benefits may warrant the use of the drug in pregnant women, despite its potential risks.

CATEGORY X

Studies in animals or humans have demonstrated fetal abnormalities, and/or positive evidence of human fetal risk exists, based on adverse reaction data from investigational or marketing experience. The risks involved with the use of the drug in pregnant women clearly outweigh its potential benefits.

*Pregnancy categories from *Mosby's drug reference for health professions,* ed 4, St Louis, 2014, Mosby/Elsevier.

Later the same day, the patient brings in another new prescription from her dentist for penicillin. When trying to enter this prescription, a DUR warning appears because the prescription signifies a ***therapeutic class duplication***. The system generates this DUR because the amoxicillin entered earlier is in the same class of medications as penicillin, and the profile information was compared. Again, the technician alerts the pharmacist, and, in this case, a call to the dentist will be made to discuss the prescription.

```
                        Dr. Elsa Valdez          Date:    2/20/2017
                       6425 W. Cedar Street
                       Cambridge, MA 02139
                       Office: (617) 555-0046
                       Fax: (617) 555-0045
    ─────────────────────────────────────────────────────────────

    Patient Name:   Karen Anderson

    Address:    526 Maple Street, Waltham, MA 02354
    R
     X          Penicillin VK 250 mg
                 1 po bid x 3 days #8

    Refill:   0

    DEA: FV1234070                              Dr. E. Valdez
                                                          M.D.
```

▪ Lab Objectives

In this Lab, you will:

- Enter given information into the database for a patient, which provides a complete profile and patient history.
- Demonstrate the ability to perform the tasks if and when a DUR warning is generated during the data-entry process.

▪ Scenario

You are continuing to work in the simulated community lab and are processing prescriptions, having added the function of reviewing and preparing a complete profile. This scenario will require entering some profile data, as well as inputting prescriptions, adding notes, and putting prescriptions on file (hold). You may refer to previous Labs 3, 6, and 9, since these tasks were practiced in earlier Labs.

▪ Pre Lab Information

You have learned all the steps to the basic functions in a community setting from previous Labs. Now the additional steps of adding diseases, allergies, notes, or diet information to a patient's profile will be performed.

▪ Student Directions

Estimated completion time: 20 minutes

1. Read through the steps in the Lab before performing the Lab exercise.
2. After reading through the Lab, perform the required steps to create a label and prepare the product for dispensing.
3. Complete the exercise at the end of the Lab.

STEPS TO ADD INFORMATION TO A PATIENT'S PROFILE AND PROCESSING A PRESCRIPTION WITH A DUR WARNING

1. Access the main screen of Visual SuperScript.

2. Click on **FILL RX'S** located on the left side of the menu screen. The *Prescription Processing* form appears.

3. Click on the **NEW RX** icon on the top left of the *Prescription Processing* form.

   Note: Prescription information such as the **RX NO.** (prescription number) and **DISPENSE DATE** are automatically generated and added to the form. You may also choose the **RX ORIGIN** from the drop-down menu if the prescription is not written.

> ▶ **LAB TIP**
>
> Enter your initials in the *Enter Tech Init* box if it does not automatically prepopulate, and click **OK**.

4. Tab to the next data field. This is the **CUSTOMER LOOKUP** text box. Type the first three letters of the customer's last name, and hit **ENTER**.

   Type *FRA* for Franks, Cynthia. Validate the DOB: 4.14.56

Dr. John Thompson
81 Highland Street
Allston, MA 02134
Office: (617) 632-4568
Fax: (617) 734-6340

Date: _____11/21/2017_____

Patient Name: ___Cynthia Franks___

Address: ___24 Willow Avenue, Allston, MA 02134___

℞ *Coumadin 5 mg 1 tab po qd #30*
    Brand necessary

Refill: ___3___

DEA: AT427831
State License: 3445542

Dr. J. Thompson
                    M.D.

---

5. Select the appropriate customer by double-clicking on the customer name or by clicking **OK** when the customer name is highlighted in blue.

   Note: The customer's personal information such as **ADDRESS**, **PHONE**, and **BIRTHDATE** will be automatically added to the *Prescription Processing* form.

   Note: You are automatically directed to the **DOCTOR** text box once the patient information is populated. For new prescriptions, the system will search the patient's prescription file to find the name of the prescriber of the most recently filled prescription. If found, then the system will insert the prescriber's name into this field.

LAB TIP

If a different physician has written the new prescription, then you can delete the old name and enter the new one.

Refer to your sample prescription and use Dr. J. Thompson.

6. Press the **Tab** key. You will be prompted to the **Prescribed Drug** data entry field. Type the first three letters of the prescribed drug into the **Prescribed Drug** data entry field. Then press **Enter**.

Enter Cou, for Coumadin 5 mg.

7. Select the appropriate drug from the *Drug Name Lookup* dialog box by double-clicking on the drug name.

8. Since the prescription states, "Brand necessary," choose **COUMADIN**, and not the generic choice.

9. A DUR warning for pregnancy will appear , as shown below. After receiving approval from the instructor (simulated pharmacist review) to continue, click **Close** to move through the warnings.

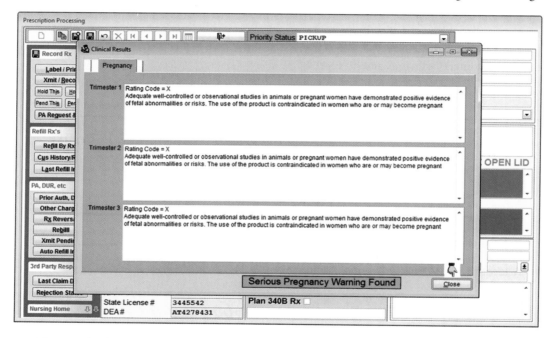

10. Use your keyboard's up and down arrows to highlight the drug option you want. Press **Enter**, and full drug information appears below, along with an image, if applicable. Choose the generic substitution unless the physician has specified dispense as written (DAW).

11. Next, you will be prompted to the **Refills Ordered** data entry field.

Key in the appropriate number of refills.

12. Press the **Tab** key. You will be prompted to enter the **Prescribed Quantity**.

*Key in the appropriate quantity in the **Prescribed Quantity** data entry field.*

13. In the **DAW** text box, choose the correct **DAW** code by clicking on the arrow on the right side of the **DAW** data entry field.

Click on the correct DAW code from the drop-down menu.

Note: When filling a prescription, knowing the correct **DAW** code to be assigned to a prescription is necessary for reimbursement. To accomplish this, distinguish between the brand name and the generic name of the medication. Although the prescriber may write the brand name of a drug on a patient's prescription, it may not necessarily mean that the brand-name drug must be dispensed. If the prescriber indicates **DAW** or "brand name medically necessary" on the patient's prescription for a brand-name drug, then the brand-name drug rather than the generic alternative MUST be dispensed. This situation, for example, would be a **DAW** code 1. Failure to use the proper **DAW** code may result in improper third-party reimbursement to the pharmacy. Seven **DAW** codes are used in the pharmacy practice:

DAW 0—Prescriber has approved the dispensing of a generic medication.
DAW 1—Prescriber requests that the brand-name drug be dispensed.
DAW 2—Prescriber has approved the dispensing of a generic drug, but the patient has requested that the brand-name drug be dispensed.
DAW 3—Pharmacist dispenses the drug as written.
DAW 4—No generic drugs are available in the store.
DAW 5—Brand-name drug is dispensed but is priced as a generic drug.
DAW 6—Registered pharmacist (RPh)–prescriber call is attempted.

14. Press the **TAB** key. Type the patient abbreviated directions in the **SIG** text box.

Key in *1T D PO* as the shortcut abbreviation S<small>IG</small>
for "Take one tablet once daily by mouth."

Note: What appears in the blue **S<small>IG</small> IN E<small>NGLISH</small>** space is what will appear on the label. If an error is made when typing in the **S<small>IG</small>**, then backspace to delete the error and retype the correct information.

15. Press the **TAB** key. You will be prompted to enter **P<small>RESCRIBED</small> D<small>AYS</small> S<small>UPPLY</small>**. Type in the appropriate days' supply in the **P<small>RESCRIBED</small> D<small>AYS</small> S<small>UPPLY</small>** data entry field.

Enter *30* for the **P<small>RESCRIBED</small> D<small>AYS</small> S<small>UPPLY</small>**

 LAB TIP

Days' supply involves calculating the number of days that a particular prescription will last. All third-party payers require this information. Failure to provide the prescribed days' supply information properly may result in the pharmacy losing money. To calculate the days' supply that a prescription will last, use the following formula:

$$\text{Days' supply} = \frac{\text{Total quantity dispensed}}{\text{Total quantity taken per day}}$$

The days' supply is the number of days a medication will last for one filling. Days' supply does not take into account refills. The majority of the third-party payers will reimburse a pharmacy for a 30-day supply of a medication.

Note: In the **R<small>X</small> N<small>OTES</small>** section, you add any notes that apply. Most states require patients to receive the opportunity for medication counseling. The **R<small>X</small> N<small>OTES</small>** section is a good place to document "any other important information".

16. Press the **ENTER** key. Click the **SAVE** 💾 icon, and note the prescription number.

17. Click on the **X<small>MIT</small>/R<small>ECORD</small>** on the left side of the screen to complete adjudication. The screen will clear and prepare to fill a new prescription. Click **LABEL/PRINT**, enter the prescription number noted previously, and print the label after verifying information.

18. For this exercise, print the prescription label, prepare the medication for dispensing, and include the stock bottle for a final check by the instructor or pharmacist.

 TECH NOTE

As a medication safety practice, verify that the image reflects the medication chosen along with NDC number.

LAB 9

Obtaining a Refill Authorization

■ Introduction

Prescriptions are written or called in for different reasons. Most often, they are written during a routine physician's office visit or after being discharged from a hospital or clinic, before or after a procedure or surgery, or when a patient calls their physician to obtain a medication, such as an antibiotic, for an acute illness. If a patient is prescribed a *maintenance* or routine medication for a *chronic* illness, such as diabetes or heart disease, then these medications are often written with refills until a follow-up or return appointment time is scheduled in 6 months, for example. The patient may be required to complete blood work or tests before his or her next visit.

MEDICATION SAFETY CONSIDERATION

If the medication is a Schedule 2 substance (CII drug), **no refills** are authorized. The patient must get a NEW written prescription from his or her physician.

If the prescriptions somehow get off schedule and the patient needs more to last until his or her next appointment, then the physician can either approve a refill if requested or ask the patient to return for an earlier appointment.

This process is called obtaining a *refill authorization* and is requested by the pharmacy as a courtesy to the customer. Most often, the turnaround time is between 24 and 48 hours, because most physician offices work on these requests at the end of the day.

The following is an example:

Customer A calls to request a refill on her furosemide (Lasix), but no refills are authorized on the prescription in the patient's profile. The technician can print a form to send to the prescriber's office to request authorization for the patient. Once approved, the prescription is sent back to the pharmacy, and the technician can create a new prescription, using the same directions and drug, as well as filling the medication for the patient. The prescriber can choose to write a prescription for 1 month to last until a scheduled appointment or, if the patient is stable, possibly longer. Whichever the case, the patient now has a NEW prescription that starts with the date of the authorization.

■ Lab Objectives

In this Lab, you will:

- Discuss the refill authorization process and the technician's role in the process.
- Demonstrate how to print a refill authorization form received via an electronic request, a written request, or a telephone call.
- Process a returned refill authorization, once approved, and create a new prescription from an expired prescription.
- Learn the procedure for faxing or scanning the prescriber for additional refill requests using an approved document.

■ Pre Lab Information

1. Access the main screen of Visual SuperScript.
2. Click on **OPTIONS** on the top right of the menu screen, and select **WORKSTATION SETUP**. Make sure your printer is selected in the **LABEL PRINTER** field.

■ Student Directions

Estimated completion time: 20 minutes

1. Read through the steps in the Lab before performing the Lab exercise.
2. After reading through the Lab, perform the required steps for a refill, or prepare a *Refill Authorization* request.
3. Answer the questions at the end of the Lab.
4. Complete the exercise at the end of the Lab.

STEPS FOR REFILLING A PRESCRIPTION USING A PRESCRIPTION NUMBER OR THE PATIENT'S NAME

1. Click the **FILL Rx's** button on the left side of the main menu. Enter the following prescription from Dr. J. Kennedy. Save and **XMIT/RECORD**.

    Larry Jones, Celebrex 100 mg, no refills, take 1 PO qd.

 LAB TIP

You will need the prescription number to complete this lab. You can either note the number or look it up by the **CUS HISTORY/REFILL** button on the left side of the screen.

2. The *Prescription Processing* dialog box appears on your screen. Click on the **REFILL BY Rx#** button located on the left side of the screen.

3. Key in the prescription number that is to be refilled in the **Rx No.** box.

4. The *Cannot Refill, Select Copy Options* dialog box appears. This dialog box will appear when a prescription has no refills remaining or if the prescription has expired.

Cannot Refill, Select Copy Options

Rx # 186542	Ph. Initials CB/RM
Prescription Date 05/10/2017	

JONES, LARRY   Customer
Birthdate 01/01/1901

Drug   CELEBREX 100 MG CAPSULE
Refills Authorized 0   Days Supply 30
Quantity 30.000   DAW Code 0
Remaining Qty 0.000

Doctor   KENNEDY, J.
Address 1623 CAMELOT DRIVE
City BRIGHTON   State MA
State License # 2556321
DEA# AK6321892   Fax (617) 439-8802
Off Phone 1 (617) 439-8800   Ext
eMail Address Dr_KENNEDY@J._KENNEDY_MD.com
SPI   Select Different SPI

Add to Fax Que
eMail Refill Request
eMail to Fax Refill Request
Fax Refill Auth Request Form
Print Refill Auth Request Form
Preview Refill Auth Request Form

☑ Process only this Rx

Sig
TK 1C QD

Date Fax to be Sent On   05/10/2017 09:53:14 AM
TAKE 1 CAPSULE ONCE DAILY

Copy to New Rx   Abort Refill

Electronic Refill Request

Preview Electronic Refill Request

DAW
0- No DAW

Rx Notes

Additional Notes

Rx #	Doctor	Customer	Drug	Quantity

Queued Fax Notes

Delete Queued Fax Request

MEDICATION SAFETY CONSIDERATION

A technician may process a refill once the authorization form is returned from the physician, and this document becomes a new prescription with the new date (as long as **no changes** have occurred). However, if the office returns the call regarding the request and has made any changes, for example, taking 2 tablets a day when the patient was taking 1, then this is now considered a **NEW** prescription, and a **PHARMACIST** must take the order.

5. Click on the green **COPY TO NEW RX** button located on the right side of the dialog box and the *Prescription Processing* dialog box will appear. If the physician has approved additional refills, then tab to the *Refill Ordered* field and complete the refill.

QUESTIONS FOR REVIEW

1. A refill authorization request was sent for Ernest Hatcher, and the nurse is on the phone with a response. A refill authorization has been requested for *Risperdal 4 mg, take 1 daily*; however, the prescriber wants to make a change and is now authorizing *Risperdal 4 mg, 2 mg at bedtime*. How should a technician handle this situation?

2. After arriving at work yesterday and listening to your telephone messages, you requested a refill for a patient at 0800. The patient calls today at 10 AM and wants to know if it is ready. What should you say?

EXERCISE

Follow the steps from the preceding Lab to process the refill authorizations for the following medication orders. Submit the labels and prepared medications for verification.

MEDICATION SAFETY CONSIDERATION

Some requests may provide only a name or prescription number with a drug name or verification of the patient by birthday or address. You MUST be sure you have the right medication and the right patient; therefore question any missing information you may need.

For example: Mr. Jones called in for his Lasix. However, he has a very common last name, and you found six Jones in your system. Request a date of birth (DOB), physician name, address, or some information to ensure you have the right patient before processing a refill request. In your class-simulated lab, the patient can be your instructor.

- WALK IN request from Brian Davidson (DOB: 2.22.76) for Ceftin 186526
- CALL IN for Cynthia Franks (DOB: 4.14.56) for Coumadin 5 mg
- CALL IN from J. Busch (DOB: 10.23.70) for Prilosec and Glucophage 500 mg *Must verify the first name because only an initial was provided.*
- CALL IN for Nancy Davis (DOB: 12.14.71) for her Ventolin inhaler.

LAB 10

Processing a Prior Authorization

▪ Introduction

Third-party companies have a list of approved medications called a *formulary*. This group of medications has been reviewed for cost, effectiveness, and therapeutic indications. When a physician prescribes a medication that is not in the formulary or is a *nonpreferred drug*, then the insurance company may require additional documentation as to the reason this specific medication is needed over a similar one found in the formulary. It may also be that the medication being prescribed is for an alternate indication, such as cosmetics or smoking cessation, which is not a disease or treatment normally covered by insurance. If the physician can justify the need, then often the drug will be covered.

▪ Lab Objectives

In this Lab, you will:

- Demonstrate the ability to perform computer functions necessary to enter a new prescription into a pharmacy system for a drug requiring prior approval including prescription interpretation, calculations, and pharmacology.
- Understand what prior drug approval or nonformulary drugs require for processing.
- Perform the necessary documentation required for prior drug approval.

▪ Scenario

You are working together in the simulated community lab and are performing the functions of processing prescriptions, requesting prior authorizations to the list, entering required data, placing prescriptions on hold, interpreting prescriptions, and completing paperwork to be sent to a physician's office. Although these tasks were practiced in earlier Labs, refer back if necessary. Use the drug reference for these exercises to find the information needed for processing each prescribed medication.

▪ Pre Lab Information

You have learned all the steps to the basic functions in a community setting from previous Labs. You will continue to work in a simulated community lab setting and complete prior authorizations. Once the prescription has been entered into the patient's profile, the documentation process can be done online, as well as manually, and is part of the adjudication process. (For this exercise, it will be completed manually and checked by your instructor). The turnaround time for this process is usually 24 to 48 hours; the patient should be made aware of this time frame. This Lab explains the steps involved in filling a new prescription for a current prior drug approval.

▪ Student Directions

1. Read through the steps in the Lab before performing the Lab exercise.
2. After reading through the Lab, perform the required steps to create a label and prepare the product for dispensing.
3. Complete the exercise at the end of the Lab.

 LAB TIP

Understanding the steps of adding a new prescription (see Lab 6) is essential before completing the following Lab.

Dr. Jonathan Crusoe
4939 W. Fir Street
Fairhaven, MA 02719
Office: (508) 555-3644
Fax: (508) 555-3646

Date: ___11/21/2017___

Patient Name: __Millie Agner__

Address: __300 S. Alder Street, Deerfield, MA 01342__

Rx

Celebrex 100 mg, 1 bid #60
Brand necessary

Refill: __0__

DEA: AK6321892
State License: 2556321

Dr. J. Crusoe
M.D.

Use the above prescription to complete the following steps.

1. Access the main screen of Visual SuperScript.

2. Click on **FILL Rx's** located on the left side of the menu screen. The *Prescription Processing* form appears.

3. Click on the **NEW Rx** icon on the top left of the *Prescription Processing* form.

   Note: Prescription information such as the **Rx No.** (prescription number) and **DISPENSE DATE** are automatically generated and added to the form. You may also choose the **Rx ORIGIN** from the drop-down menu if the prescription is not written.

> ▷ **LAB TIP**
>
> Enter your initials in the *Enter Tech Init* box if it appears, and click **OK**.

4. Tab to the next field. This is the **CUSTOMER LOOKUP** (highlighted in blue) data entry field. Type the first three letters of the customer's last name, and hit **ENTER**.

   Type *AGN* for Agner, Millie.

   Validate the DOB (11.06.1929).

5. Select the appropriate customer by double-clicking on the customer name or by clicking **OK** when the customer name is highlighted in blue.

   Note: The customer's personal information such as **ADDRESS**, **PHONE**, and **BIRTHDATE** will be automatically added to the *Prescription Processing* form.

Note: You are automatically directed to the **Doctor** text box once the patient information is populated. For new prescriptions, the system will search the patient's prescription file to find the name of the prescriber of the most recently filled prescription. If found, then the system will insert the prescriber's name into this field. If a different physician has written the new prescription, then you can delete the old name and enter the new one. For this particular exercise, the physician, Dr. J. Crusoe, is listed in the sample prescription. If the doctor's information is not automatically populated in this field, then refer to your sample prescription and use Dr. J. Crusoe.

6. Press the **Tab** key. You will be prompted to the **Prescribed Drug** data entry field. Type the first three letters of the prescribed drug into the **Prescribed Drug** data entry field. Then press **Enter**.

Enter Cel for Celebrex 100 mg.

7. Select the appropriate drug from the list in the *Drug Name Lookup* dialog box by double-clicking on the drug name.

 LAB TIP

If a series of warning dialog boxes appear, these are known as drug utilization reviews (DURs). The patient's medication history is compared against the drug you are entering for pregnancy warnings, drug-drug and drug-food interactions, or contraindication conditions or diseases. (The warning messages should be viewed and approved by the pharmacist before dispensing the medication.)

---

8. After receiving approval from the instructor (simulated pharmacist review) to continue, click the **Close** icon to move through the warnings.

9. Brand and generic drugs will appear under the heading *Available Drug Choices*. Use your keyboard's up and down keys to highlight the drug option you want. Press **Enter** and full drug information appears below, along with an image if available. Choose the generic substitution unless the physician has specified dispense as written (DAW).

10. Next, you will be prompted to the **Refills Ordered** data entry field.

Key in the appropriate number of refills.

11. Press the **Tab** key. You will be prompted to enter the **Prescribed Quantity**.

Key in the appropriate quantity in the **Prescribed Quantity** data entry field.

12. In the **DAW** text box. Choose the correct **DAW** code by clicking on the arrow on the right side of the **DAW** data entry field.

Click on the correct DAW code from the drop-down menu.

Note: When filling a prescription, knowing the correct **DAW** code to be assigned to a prescription is necessary for reimbursement. To accomplish this, distinguish between the brand name and the generic name of the medication. Although the prescriber may write the brand name of a drug on a patient's prescription, it may not necessarily mean that the brand-name drug must be dispensed. If the prescriber indicates **DAW** or "brand name medically necessary" on the patient's prescription for a brand-name drug, then the brand-name drug rather than the generic alternative MUST be dispensed. This situation, for example, would be a **DAW** code 1. Failure to use the proper **DAW** code may result in improper third-party reimbursement to the pharmacy. Seven **DAW** codes are used in the pharmacy practice:

DAW 0—Prescriber has approved the dispensing of a generic medication.

DAW 1—Prescriber requests that the brand-name drug be dispensed.

DAW 2—Prescriber has approved the dispensing of a generic drug, but the patient has requested that the brand-name drug be dispensed.

DAW 3—Pharmacist dispenses the drug as written.

DAW 4—No generic drugs are available in the store.

DAW 5—Brand-name drug is dispensed but is priced as a generic drug.

DAW 6—Registered pharmacist (RPh)–prescriber call is attempted.

13. Press the **TAB** key. Type the patient abbreviated directions in the **SIG** text box.

> **Key in *1C BID PO* as the shortcut abbreviation SIG for "Take one capsule twice daily by mouth."**

Note: What appears in the blue **SIG IN ENGLISH** space is what will appear on the label. If an error is made when typing in the **SIG**, then backspace to delete the error and retype the correct information.

14. Press the **TAB** key. You will be prompted to enter **PRESCRIBED DAYS SUPPLY**. Type in the appropriate days' supply in the **PRESCRIBED DAYS SUPPLY** data entry field.

> **Enter *30* for the PRESCRIBED DAYS SUPPLY.**

 LAB TIP

Days' supply involves calculating the number of days that a particular prescription will last. All third-party payers require this information. Failure to provide the prescribed days' supply information properly may result in the pharmacy losing money. To calculate the days' supply that a prescription will last, use the following formula:

$$\text{Days' supply} = \frac{\text{Total quantity dispensed}}{\text{Total quantity taken per day}}$$

The days' supply is the number of days a medication will last for one filling. Days' supply does not take into account refills. The majority of the third-party payers will reimburse a pharmacy for a 30-day supply of a medication.

Note: You may tab back to the **RX NOTES** section and add any notes that apply. Most states require patients to receive the opportunity for medication counseling. The **RX NOTES** section is a good place to document "offered counseling, but patient refused counseling" or other important information. Enter the following note: "Prior-approved drug request sent to physician, dated, and with your initials."

15. Press the **ENTER** key, and then click the **SAVE** 💾 icon.

16. Click on **XMIT/RECORD** on the left of the screen, and the following screen will appear, rejecting the transmission because it requires prior authorization. Click **CLOSE**.

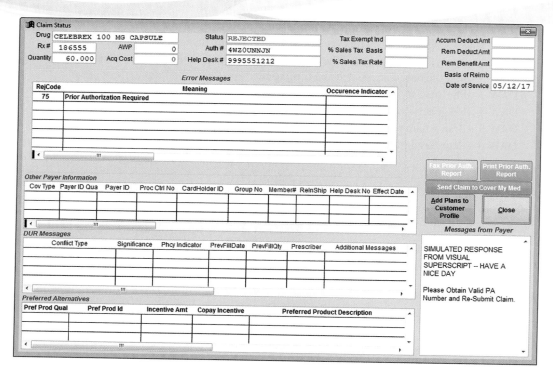

17. The *Claim Rejected* dialog box will appear. Choose **MAKE CHANGES AND RESUBMIT**.

18. From the *Prescription Processing* dialog box, choose **PRIOR AUTH, DUR** from the left side of the screen.

19. The *Prior Authorization, DUR, etc* dialog box appears. Enter the following:

> Enter the number 1 in the *Prior Auth Code* data entry field.
> Enter the number 7 a total of 11 times in the *Prior Auth #* data entry field.

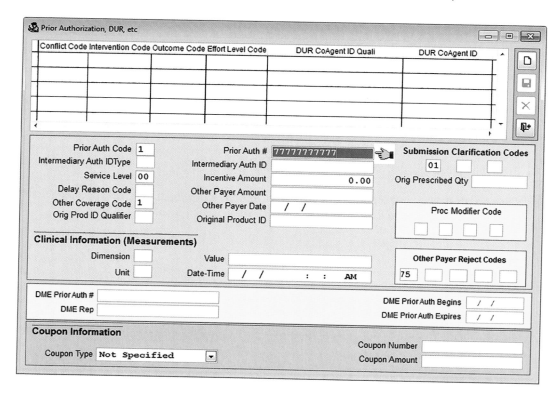

20. Click the **CLOSE** ⏻ icon near the top right of the screen, then **SAVE** 💾 , and finally **XMIT/RECORD**. The screen should show that the claim was paid.

21. Manually complete the Pharmacy section only of the *Prior Authorization* (PA) form for this drug.

22. A copy of the PA form, the prescription, and the pharmacy label will be filed until the PA form is returned with approval, usually in 24 to 48 hours. Once the approval is granted, the prescription can be filled for the patient.

23. For this exercise, print the prescription label and prepare the PA form for your instructor to check.

EXERCISE

Enter prescriptions and prepare a separate PA form for each of the following prescriptions , using the prescription and blank PA forms given to you by your instructor.

Dr. James Furman
3345 Atrium Drive
Albany, NY 12205
Office: (518) 555-4677
Fax: (518) 555-4679

Date: ___11/21/2017___

Patient Name: __Sammy Gainer__

Address: __1034 N. Laurel Street, Lexington, MA 02421__

℞ *Aciphex 20 mg 1 qd #30*
Brand necessary

Refill: __2__

DEA: AF5190688

Dr. J. Furman
M.D.

Dr. Hernando Reyes
5535 W. Cedar Street
Cambridge, MA 02139
(617) 555-9247
Fax: (617) 555-9249

Date: ___11/21/2017___

Patient Name: __Kinley Abston__

Address: __201 Maple Street, Cambridge, MA 02139-1234__

℞ *Otezla 30 mg, 1 qd #30*
Brand necessary

Refill: __0__

DEA: FR1234412

Dr. H. Reyes
M.D.

Dr. Stephanie Wrangler
1700 W. Willow Street
Westwood, MA 02090
Office: (781) 555-3012
Fax: (781) 555-3014

Date: _11/21/2017_

Patient Name: _Otis Kearns_

Address: _5028 W. Cedar Street, Cambridge, MA 02139_

℞

Movantik 25 mg 1 qd #30
If not tolerated, reduce to 12.5 mg qd
Brand necessary

Refill: _3_

DEA: BW1234828

Dr. S. Wrangler
M.D.

Dr. Karl Kalcevic
901 Mahagony Street
Marshfield, MA 02050
Office: (781) 555-6432
(781) 555-6434

Date: _11/21/2017_

Patient Name: _Natalia Acevedo_

Address: _1708 N. Hickory Street, Kingston, MA 02364_

℞

Jardiance 10 mg 1 qAM #30
Brand necessary

Refill: _0_

Dr. K. Kalcevic
M.D.

Leave all documentation, the original prescription, and the prepared label for a final check by the pharmacist.

Note: Practice using the abbreviation shortcuts found in Sig Abbreviations chart in the front of the book to make the data entry process quicker. All drug community software programs use these abbreviations to save time. Some prescriptions may require adding new patient information, new prescriber information, or adding a new drug to the database. You may review previous Labs for these procedures.

 LAB TIP

Use your drug reference for dosages, special handling (e.g., refrigeration), and drug classification.

LAB 11

Refilling, Transferring, Filling, and Prescription Reversal

■ Introduction

In the community setting, customers want the flexibility to have a prescription *filled* or *refilled* at different locations. Sometimes the location may be a completely different business, or it may be just another location of the same company. One benefit of working in a *CHAIN* or *FRANCHISE* system is that information can be shared, in some cases, between stores and states. A patient's prescription history or profile may be accessed between stores in case the patient chooses to get a prescription filled at a different location. For refills, patients may ask to process an existing medication by supplying an old bottle, prescription number, or drug name and the store where it was last filled. Each state has certain regulations that dictate whether a medication can be transferred in and out of a state, and these regulations must be followed. If transfers are allowed, specific information must be shared between the corresponding pharmacies.

MEDICATION SAFETY CONSIDERATION

Knowing your state rules and the medications and their classifications is essential to being a successful technician. When in doubt, ASK!

Another common task performed on a daily basis is the reversal of charges. If a patient chooses not to get a medication, perhaps because of cost or that they have excess at home, then the prescription can be reversed; that is, the charge that was sent to the insurance company is taken out of the system. There are even instances during which the patient may decide to pay cash when he or she comes in to pick up the medication, instead of processing it through a third-party payer. As a result, the prescription charges sent to the insurance company will need to be reversed and changed to *CASH*.

 LAB TIP

Always review the patient's profile for billing and insurance information, and ask the patient, if he or she is in your store, whether any changes have occurred. This will save valuable time if the correct billing preference and insurance information is verified and correctly charged the first time.

Another common function in a community pharmacy practice is "putting a prescription **on HOLD**." For example, a patient goes to the physician for a routine 6-month visit to check for diabetes management. If he or she leaves with a new set of prescriptions and takes this new set to the drug store that still has existing refills on the last set of prescriptions, then the new set of prescriptions can be entered into the patient's profile and placed on *HOLD*. These prescriptions can be saved and filled at a later date once the refills on the older prescriptions are used up.

MEDICATION SAFETY CONSIDERATION

Older patients will often ask to have their prescriptions placed on HOLD so that they are not lost or stolen, which will ensure that they always have a current supply of medications on hand.

■ Lab Objectives

In this Lab, you will:

- Process a customer's set of refilled prescriptions with the remaining refills that are on file; the refills may be phoned in, electronically submitted, or personally brought in by hand.
- Perform the computer functions to transfer a prescription to another pharmacy.
- Complete the steps to put a prescription on file.
- Process a prescription reversal.

■ Scenario

Today is a busy day at your simulated pharmacy, and you have learned almost all the functions of data entry through previous Lab exercises. Working as a team, assign someone to data entry, front counter, phone, inventory, and processing (counting and pouring). Use the tech-check-tech (TCT) system to check each other's work, or ask questions as you work through the day's activities.

■ Pre Lab Information

Review all the Labs to date, and have your book ready if you need to review as you are working through the tasks. In some cases, you will print screens for verification of a completed task, and then actual labels and bottles will be prepared for checking by the pharmacist (your instructor). Carefully read the directions for each exercise before beginning.

■ Student Directions

Estimated completion time: 60 minutes

1. Read through the steps in each of the Lab exercises before performing the Lab exercise.
2. After reading through the Lab, perform the required steps to complete the tasks in each scenario.

REFILLING PRESCRIPTIONS BY CUSTOMER NAME

Scenario

Mr. Ronald Jackson asks you to refill all of his medications for January and February, 2017. He may not remember all of the names or all of his prescription numbers. You can use the customer profile to locate each one for refilling.

Task

Fill Ronald Jackson's 2017 medications.

MEDICATION SAFETY CONSIDERATION

Remember the five rights—especially the right medication and the right patient. What will you ask him while you are reviewing the profile to ensure that you have the right medication and the right patient?

STEPS TO REFILL RONALD JACKSON'S 2017 MEDICATIONS

Use the information in the previous scenario to complete the following steps.

1. Access the main screen of Visual SuperScript.

2. Click on **FILL RX'S** located on the left side of the menu screen. The *Prescription Processing* form appears.

3. Click on **CUS HISTORY/REFILL**.

4. Type the customer name into the **CUSTOMER** data entry field. Press the **ENTER** key. The *Customer Lookup* dialog box will appear. Click on the correct customer from the list in the *Customer Lookup* dialog box. Click **OK**.

Enter JAC for Jackson, Ronald.

5. Select the tab titled **PRESCRIPTIONS ON FILE**. Put a checkmark in the check box of the prescriptions that need to be refilled. For this exercise, we will refill all active prescriptions (inactive prescriptions are grayed out).

6. Click on **FILL RX** located at the top of the dialog box.

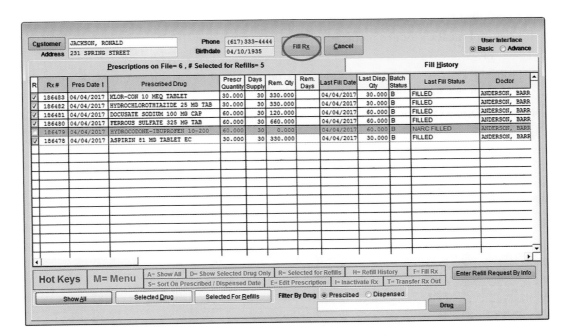

Note: If the prescription has not expired and refills are remaining, then the *Prescription Processing* form is updated with the refill information and a label can be printed.

Note: If the prescription has expired or has no refills, then follow the procedure in Lab 7 for obtaining a *Refill Authorization* request.

7. The *Prescription Processing* form now returns to the screen. All medications checked will be processed. Click on **XMIT/RECORD** located at the top left of the form. Clicking on **LABEL/PRINT** will prompt the software to adjudication.

TRANSFERRING A PRESCRIPTION

Scenario

Mrs. Shirley Jones telephones the pharmacy explaining that she is on vacation visiting her daughter in Chicago, Illinois. Mrs. Jones is out of her Hyzaar. She requests that you give her Hyzaar prescription information to a nearby pharmacy in Chicago that would enable her to refill her medication.

Task

Follow the "Steps to Transferring a Prescription" listed below to transfer Shirley Jones' prescription for Hyzaar to the following pharmacy:

Sutcliffe Pharmacy
801 West Irving Park Road
Chicago, IL 60613
Phone: (773) 525-0081
Fred Fixit, RPh

STEPS TO TRANSFERRING A PRESCRIPTION

Use the information in the above scenario to complete the following steps.

1. Access the main screen of Visual SuperScript.

2. Click on **FILL RX'S** located on the left side of the menu screen. The *Prescription Processing* form will appear.

3. From the *Prescription Processing* form, click on the arrow to scroll down to **MISC** (miscellaneous) located on the bottom left corner of the form.

4. Click on **XFER OUT** (transfer out). The *Customer History: Transfer Rx Out* dialog box will appear.

5. Key in the customer's name in the **CUSTOMER** data entry field. Press the **ENTER** key. The *Customer Lookup* dialog box will appear. Click on the appropriate customer from the lookup list, and click **OK**.

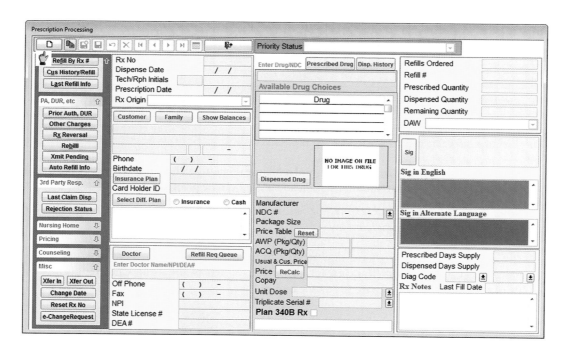

6. Put a checkmark in the checkbox of the prescription that should be transferred to another pharmacy.

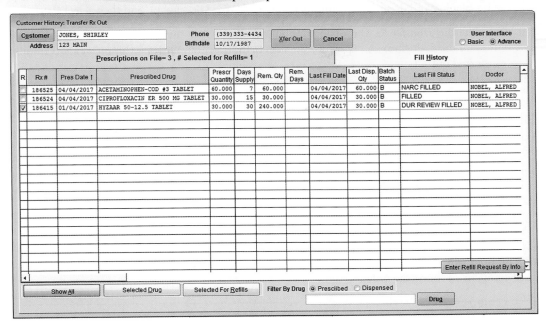

7. Click on **Xfer Out** located at the top of the dialog box, which will create a record of the transferred prescription in the patient's profile.

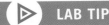

LAB TIP

At this time, the pharmacist or pharmacy technician at the pharmacy (depending on the state laws) will call the pharmacy to which the prescription is being transferred. Certain information is required, and **many states require a pharmacist, only, to transfer prescriptions and to accept transferred prescriptions**. You may need to enter the pharmacy contact information (address and phone number) before you can transfer the prescription.

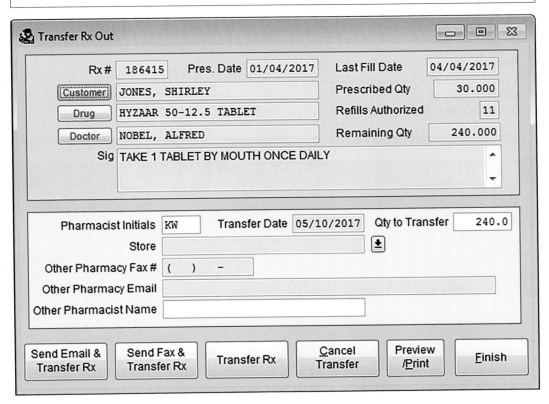

8. Print the screen by using the **Prnt Scrn** option on your keyboard. Press the **Prnt Scrn** key, open a blank Word document, right-click the blank Word document, and then select **Paste**.

9. Complete the *Transfer Rx Out* dialog box information. Click on **Transfer Rx** located at the bottom of the dialog box. A dialog box appears to indicate that the prescription was successfully transferred out.

PUTTING A PRESCRIPTION ON FILE

Scenario

Mrs. Carla Watson is at the pharmacy this afternoon with two prescriptions from her dentist. One prescription is for an antibiotic, and the other is for blood pressure medication. Mrs. Watson would like to have the prescription for the antibiotic filled, but she is sure that she has enough of her blood pressure medication at home and requests not to have that one filled. She requests that you hold it until she returns home.

Task

Place Mrs. Carla Watson's prescription for blood pressure medication on hold. Placing the prescription on hold will electronically store the prescription for Mrs. Watson without charging her insurance company or filling the order.

John Burns, DDS
123 Main Street
Brighton, MA 02135
Office: (617) 456-7765
Fax: (617) 431-5320

Date: _7/7/2017_

Patient Name: _Carla Watson_

Address: _1010 Haverford Street, Chestnut Hill, MA 02167_

  Coreg 6.25 mg bid #60

Refill: _5_

DEA: AB3623457
State License: 5432456

Dr. J. Burns
M.D.

 LAB TIP

Placing prescriptions on hold also ensures that drug-drug interactions are reviewed. This safety feature will ensure that no interactions or allergic reactions to the medication being added will occur, because the information in the patient profile is systematically reviewed each time a new drug is entered. This feature is available for over-the-counter (OTC) medications as well, if they are entered.

STEPS TO PUTTING A PRESCRIPTION ON FILE

Use the information in the scenario on the previous page to complete the following steps.

1. Access the main screen of Visual SuperScript.

2. Click on **Fill Rx's** located on the left side of the menu screen. The *Prescription Processing* form will appear.

Community Pharmacy Practice

3. From the *Prescription Processing* form, complete the patient and prescription information as you would if you were filling a new prescription. (Refer to Lab 6 for directions.)

4. After the *Prescription Processing* form is completed, click on **HOLD THIS** located at the top left corner of the form.

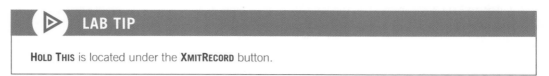

LAB TIP

HOLD THIS is located under the **XMITRECORD** button.

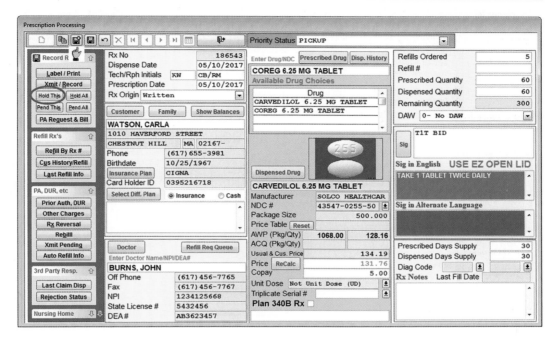

5. Although this medication will not be filled, a label will be generated. A section of the label will be filed with the prescription hard copy for record-keeping purposes.

LAB TIP

To ensure that the data was correctly entered, one of the stickers from the printed label will go on the back of the hard copy prescription before being checked by the pharmacist and filed.

6. Click on **CUS HISTORY/REFILL** located on the left side of the screen. Check to confirm that the prescription has been put on file.

7. A prescription that has been put on file or *on hold* can be filled at a later date by accessing the prescription from the customer history.

8. You have learned how to perform many fill and refill functions. Do you know how to take the prescription off hold and to return to fill it later?

9. Locate Mrs. Watson's prescription for Coreg from the customer's history. Fill the prescription.

REVERSING A PRESCRIPTION ORDER

Scenario

Carla Watson has decided that she does not need her Coreg filled. Using the **RX REVERSAL** directions, return the medication to stock, and reverse the claim to her insurance.

Use the information in the above scenario to complete the following steps.

1. Access the main screen of Visual SuperScript.

2. Click on **FILL RX'S** located on the left side of the menu screen. The *Prescription Processing* form will appear.

3. Click on the **RX REVERSAL** button on the left side of the screen.

Community Pharmacy Practice

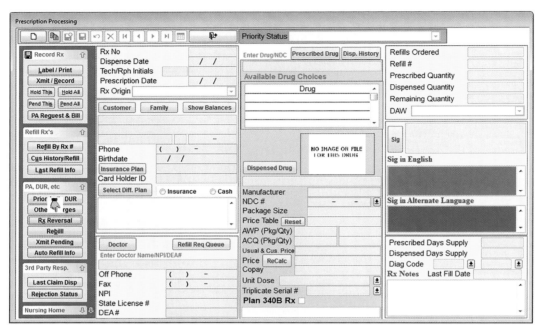

4. In the **RX REVERSAL** box, enter in the prescription number and fill date.

5. Enter in the customer's insurance information when prompted to reverse the prescription on insurance.

6. Click **PROCEED** to reverse the prescription. Continue to click **OK** or **YES** to complete the reversal.

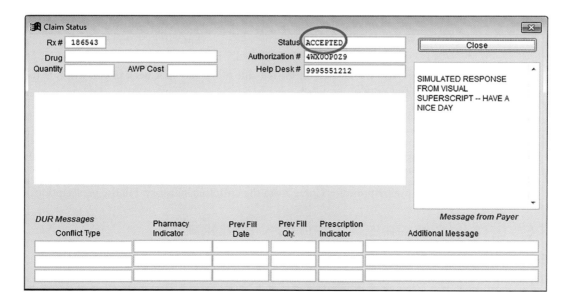

LAB 12

ePrescribing Using the eRX Feature

▪ Introduction

The community pharmacy setting is designed around dispensing *prescriptions* that are written or electronically submitted through pharmacy management systems and retained in a QUE, or electronic storage space. This transfer of prescriptions from the physician provides an extra layer of safety because the prescriptions are not handwritten, which can lead to misinterpretation. In addition, this fast transfer of information can be shared with health care professionals in real time to provide the most current profile.

In addition to the new prescriptions sent electronically, the system allows for *walk ins* and is often connected to the telephone request line for refills (interactive voice response [*IVR*]) and will also have these prescriptions loaded in the QUE for the pharmacy to fill. In a busy store, one or two technicians will often be dedicated to processing prescriptions. Prioritizing the order of processing these prescriptions is a part of the technician's duty. For instance, the first prescriptions to be processed would be WALK INS, then NEW prescriptions, and last REFILL prescriptions. Often, the data and time information for receiving and requesting a pick-up or delivery timetable is also part of the system.

▪ Lab Objectives

In this Lab, you will:

- Demonstrate how to perform necessary computer functions to enter a new prescription into a pharmacy system from the eRX system.
- Use shortcuts when entering **Sigs**.
- Apply rules for noncontrolled and controlled medications when filling and preparing them for dispensing.
- Demonstrate the technician's role in the medication use process.
- Correctly interpret and calculate prescriptions for preparation.
- Apply billing techniques to written prescriptions when performing data entry (e.g., third party, cash, Medicare/Medicaid).

▪ Scenario

You are working in a busy retail pharmacy today, and several prescriptions, which were sent in over-night through the eRX system, need to be prepared for patient pickup. Using the knowledge and data skills you have learned and performed to date, you need to enter or process each prescription, create a label or refill request if needed, and then prepare the medication by counting or pouring.

 LAB TIP

Using the shortcut abbreviations made for the software will save time, and this is very important in a busy store. See the Sig Abbreviations chart in the front of the book once you interpret the prescription and before the entry process begins. For example, typing **AP1-2GD** would be the same as having to type out "Apply 1 or 2 drops daily."

■ Pre Lab Information

Regardless of the practice setting for the pharmacy technician and pharmacist, entering data into the computer is a major component of their workload. In the retail setting, for example, a physician may electronically submit a prescription while the patient is still in his or her office, or a customer may call the refill line and request a refill with a prescription number entry. Customers will walk in and expect their requests or new prescription to be ready for them. After the pharmacy technician has retrieved the prescription from the QUE, the information is processed and the medication is counted or poured. Reviewing the steps involved in interpreting and entering a prescription is beneficial before completing the following Lab.

■ Student Directions

Estimated completion time: 1.5 hour

1. Read through the steps in the previous Labs 1 through 11 before performing the Lab exercise.
2. Using the Sig Abbreviations chart in the front of the book for abbreviations or codes, interpret the prescription directions and decide what should be typed out in the *Sig in English* field.
3. Perform the required steps to create labels and to prepare the product for dispensing.
4. Enter and prepare the prescriptions through the eRX system.

STEPS TO ENTER A NEW PRESCRIPTION

After retrieving two prescriptions from the eRX system, process both prescriptions.

1. Access the main screen of Visual SuperScript.

2. Click on the left bar at the top of the page (left side). The **QUEUED RX'S** window appears and will look similar to this.

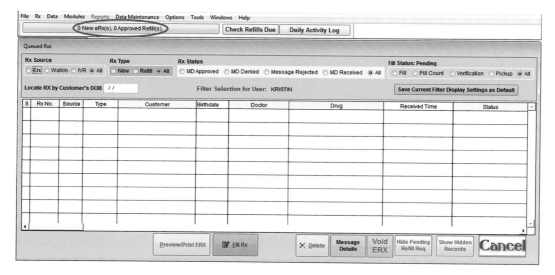

 LAB TIP

QUEUED RX'S are the prescriptions that have been electronically sent, either from a physician's office or through the refill request line from a customer entering a prescription number via the telephone. Your QUE may be different from the QUE of another student if your instructor has prefilled the information.

3. Remember to prioritize your list with WALK INS first, then NEW prescriptions, and last REFILL prescriptions, unless a special situation overrides this sequence.

4. Once the prescriptions labels are prepared and processed for prior approval or the refill request has been prepared, if needed, (see previous Labs for instructions), either count what is required or print a document or screenshot for what task is needed. For instance, if a refill request was sent, then print the form for your instructor to check.

LAB 13

Narcotic Inventory and Management

▪ Introduction

Controlled substances that are considered CII drugs are kept in a special double-locked cabinet or apart from regular stock. In addition, a perpetual inventory is kept of all Schedule II *controlled substances* or *narcotics*, which requires that each time a prescription for a CII drug is filled, the prescription is logged and the quantity is subtracted from the inventory. The prescription may be stamped with a red "C" stamp, numbered differently, and/or separately filed from all other drugs. A copy of the ordering form (Drug Enforcement Administration [DEA] 222) should be kept with the invoice for a minimum of 2 years, although regulations vary from state to state.

Each pharmacy or dispensing facility must keep accurate records of all CII drugs dispensed, and, as a pharmacy technician, you will be involved in this process under a pharmacist's supervision. Your responsibilities may include checking in a shipment, preparing returns for reverse distributors, ordering, or creating reports.

MEDICATION SAFETY CONSIDERATION

Always be aware of BOTH state and federal law updates on the duties of a technician regarding dispensing and record-keeping requirements for controlled drugs. In addition, a drug may be considered a controlled substance in your state but not necessarily at the federal level.

▪ Scenario

Today, you and a fellow student will be working together in the narcotics area of the hospital pharmacy. You will double count current stock, enter an order, and prepare a Control Drug Report.

▪ Student Directions

Estimated completion time: 45 minutes
1. Read through the steps in the Lab before performing the Lab exercise.
2. After reading through the Lab, perform the required steps to complete the tasks in the scenario.

STEPS TO PRINT A CONTROL DRUG REPORT FOR ENTRY

1. Access the main screen of Visual SuperScript.

2. Click on **REPORTS** from the menu toolbar located at the top of the screen.

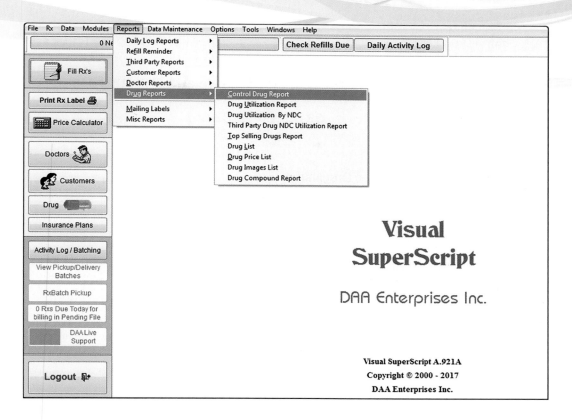

3. Select **Drug Reports** from the drop-down menu. Then select **Control Drug Report** from the expanded menu.

4. The *Control Drug Report* dialog box appears. Note that the insertion point is in the first data entry field, **Date From**.

5. **Note:** Deleting the default date that appears in the data entry field is not necessary. The date that is typed in will replace the existing default date of 6 months.

6. The **Drug Class** field will designate if the report will generate a list of Class/Schedule II drugs only: **C2 Only**; Class/Schedule III through Class/Schedule V: **C3-C5** drugs; or all the drugs in the report: **All (C2-C5)** drugs. Click on the appropriate choice.

   Select **All (C2-C5)**.

7. The **Sort by** field will designate the order in which the report should be arranged. Indicate how the report should be arranged: **Fill Date**, **Drug Name**, or **Customer**. Click on the appropriate choice.

   Select **Drug Name**.

8. Choose the appropriate **Report Layout**.

   Select Detail.

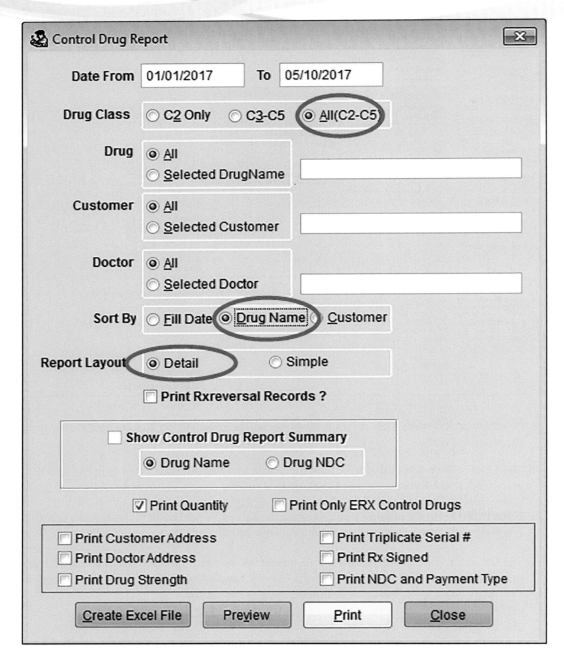

9. Click on **PREVIEW** located at the bottom of the *Control Drug Report* dialog box. The selected *Control Drug Report* will open and appear on the screen.

```
                    DAA EDUCATIONAL SOFTWARE              PAGE NO: 1/2
              369 HARVARD ST, SUITE 1,BROOKLINE, MA 02446
                         (617) 734-7366                   DATE: 05/10/17


                    Controlled Drugs Report For Sched 2-5
                           (01/01/17 To 05/10/17)


Type Rx#   OrigDate FillDate Ref   Customer          Doctor           Drug              Class Qty    RPh  DEA#          Sig
     171370 10/01/16 01/02/17 3/2  BEASON, PATRINA   LAKHANI, DEEPAK  PHENOBARBITAL 32.4 MG  C4 60.00 RM/RMBL1234931 TAKE 1 TABLET BY MOUTH TWICE DAILY
     177402 11/07/16 01/02/17 1/1  VICKERS, CAMELIA  CRUSOE, JONATHAN LYRICA 50 MG CAPSULE   C5 90.00 RM/RMFC1234068 TAKE 1 CAPSULE BY MOUTH 3 TIMES A
     177403 11/07/16 01/02/17 1/1  VICKERS, CAMELIA  CRUSOE, JONATHAN TRAMADOL HCL 50 MG     C4 90.00 RM/RMFC1234068 TAKE 1 TABLET BY MOUTH EVERY 8
     178432 11/14/16 01/02/17 0/3  DEBEERS, TERRENCE ZABARSKI, MICHAEL ALPRAZOLAM 2 MG TABLET C4 60.00 RM/RMWZ1234400 TAKE 1 TABLET BY MOUTH TWICE DAILY
     183485 12/16/16 01/02/17 1/1  SLADE, KARINA     CHAPELLE, AKHI   ACETAMINOPHEN-COD #3   C3 56.00 RM/RMFC1234258 TAKE 1 TABLET BY MOUTH EVERY 6
     184445 12/22/16 01/02/17 0/1  ADAMS, MARGARET   DOSCH, RAMEZ     LORAZEPAM 1 MG TABLET  C4 30.00 RM/RMFC1234929 TAKE 1 TABLET BY MOUTH AT BEDTIME
     185878 01/02/17 01/02/17 0/1  WHITAKER, GLORIA  CRUSOE, JONATHAN ALPRAZOLAM 2 MG TABLET C4 60.00 RM/RMFC1234068 TAKE 1 TABLET BY MOUTH EVERY 12
     185899 01/02/17 01/02/17 0/0  CARROLLTON,       CRUSOE, JONATHAN HYDROCODONE/APAP 7.5/325 C2 60.00 RM/RMFC1234068 TAKE 1 TABLET BY MOUTH EVERY 12
     185900 01/02/17 01/02/17 0/1  CARROLLTON,       CRUSOE, JONATHAN ALPRAZOLAM 2 MG TABLET C4 60.00 RM/RMFC1234068 TAKE 1 TABLET BY MOUTH TWICE DAILY
     185996 01/02/17 01/02/17 0/1  OLIVARES, MARIA   CRUSOE, JONATHAN ZOLPIDEM 10 MG TABLET  C4 30.00 RM/RMFC1234068 TAKE 1 TABLET BY MOUTH EVERY NIGHT
     179334 11/18/16 01/03/17 1/2  SMITH, RODNEY     JABRI, AYMAN     LORAZEPAM 2 MG TABLET  C4 60.00 RM/RMBJ1234397 TAKE 1 TABLET BY MOUTH TWICE DAILY
     186056 12/29/16 01/03/17 0/0  PARKHURST, BARBARA MCCLAIN, MICHELLE HYDROCODONE/APAP 7.5/325 C2 30.00 RM/RMMM1234222 TAKE 1 TABLET BY MOUTH TWICE DAILY
     186225 01/03/17 01/03/17 0/0  ANDERSON, GENE    TILLMAN, PETER   HYDROCODONE/APAP 5/325 C2 40.00 RM/RMFT1234878 TAKE 1 TABLET BY MOUTH TWICE DAILY
     186240 01/02/17 01/03/17 0/0  SANFORD, CORINE   CHIHARA, MATT    ALPRAZOLAM 0.25 MG     C4 30.00 RM/RMFC1234359 TAKE 1 TABLET BY MOUTH DAILY FOR
     186245 01/03/17 01/03/17 0/3  VENZIANO, JUANITA CRUSOE, JONATHAN TRAMADOL HCL 50 MG     C4 60.00 RM/RMFC1234068 TAKE 1 TABLET BY MOUTH EVERY 12
     186249 01/03/17 01/03/17 0/2  THERIEN, DAVID    ALBEHEARY, NAJWA ZOLPIDEM 10 MG TABLET  C4 30.00 RM/RMBA1234309 TAKE 1 TABLET BY MOUTH EVERY NIGHT
     174374 10/18/16 01/04/17 2/3  LITTLEFIELD,      AZMI, HUMA       TRAMADOL HCL 50 MG     C4 60.00 RM/RMFC1234068 TAKE 1 TABLET BY MOUTH 3 TIMES A
     181882 12/04/16 01/04/17 1/1  BISCHOFF, TOMASZ  CRUSOE, JONATHAN TRAMADOL HCL 50 MG     C4 60.00 RM/RMFC1234068 TAKE 1 TABLET BY MOUTH TWICE DAILY
     186252 01/03/17 01/04/17 0/0  SMITH, RODNEY     PASCHAL, JOSEPH  BUPRENORPHIN-NALOXON 8-2 C3 30.00 RM/RMAP1234929 PLACE 1 TABLET UNDER THE TONGUE
     186257 01/04/17 01/04/17 0/2  SOTOMAYOR, LUIS   DOSCH, RAMEZ     ALPRAZOLAM 1 MG TABLET C4 60.00 RM/RMAD1234929 TAKE 1 TABLET BY MOUTH TWICE DAILY
     186262 01/04/17 01/04/17 0/3  TOMEI, DENELLE    DOSCH, RAMEZ     ALPRAZOLAM 1 MG TABLET C4 45.00 RM/RMAD1234929 TAKE 1 TABLET BY MOUTH ONCE DAILY
     186321 01/04/17 01/04/17 0/0  DANIELSON, DARREN MAHADEO, DEEPAK  TRAMADOL HCL 50 MG     C4 30.00 RM/RMBM1234056 TAKE 1 TABLET BY MOUTH EVERY 6
     186332 01/04/17 01/04/17 0/0  CUNNINGTON, KEITH MAHADEO, DEEPAK  ACETAMINOPHEN-COD #3   C3 90.00 RM/RMBM1234056 TAKE 1 TABLET BY MOUTH EVERY 4-6
```

10. Click on the **PRINT REPORT** 🖨 icon located at the top right of the *Print Preview* toolbar.

11. Click on the **CLOSE PREVIEW** 🔚 icon located at the top right of the *Print Preview* toolbar. The report is closed out, and the *Control Drug Report* dialog box returns.

12. Verify the amounts against the report you completed to ensure that the amounts match the current inventory in the database.

13. Once completed, provide the chart and report to the instructor, indicating that the report is now ready to check.

LAB 14

Durable and Nondurable Medication Equipment and Supplies

■ Introduction

Pharmacy practice is ever changing. As a result of the implementation of the Affordable Care Act and the growing population of older adults, additional supplies and services are now being offered through the pharmacy. Many chains, franchises, and independent pharmacies offer durable medical equipment (DME) and non-DME, devices, and supplies. Typical items include the following:

- Wheelchairs, DME, and supplies
- Medical nutrition
- Infusion therapy
- Prosthetic and orthotic devices and supplies

The pharmacy technician's role does not only include prescription processing, but it also includes an understanding of disease prevention, wellness promotion, health screenings, and other factors that affect health. Smoking cessation and drug-abuse prevention are part of the approach to total care for a patient.

■ Lab Objectives

In this Lab, you will:

- Use the electronic patient profile to record and identify DME and non-DME, supplies, or devices.
- Assist the pharmacist in preparing and dispensing common DME or non-DME for dispensing.
- Understand the technician's role in wellness and disease prevention by maintaining a current patient profile and history.
- Role play in a simulated environment to answer common questions concerning DME, including quality assurance. Verify each other's work (simulate the tech-check-tech [TCT] process).

ASHP goals: 1, 3-9, 11, 13-19, 32-36, and 40-45.

■ Scenario

Today, you are working in a simulated retail setting in the DME area of the pharmacy. Requests for DME and non-DME and related supplies will be made, and some requests will require data entry of a prescription. Working in teams, you will role play customer interactions (provided by your instructor) and follow proper guidelines for interpreting, preparing, and interacting with customers.

■ Pre Lab Information

This Lab exercise will give you an opportunity to work with some common DME and non-DME and interact with other students in customer-based scenarios. You will also use the database and profiles for information and records, as well as notes required for these items.

■ Student Directions

Estimated completion time: 30 minutes

1. Read through the steps in the Lab before performing the Lab exercises.
2. After reading through the Lab, perform the required steps to prepare the DME and non-DME supplies.

STEPS FOR DISPENSING A GLUCOSE METER AND SUPPLIES

 LAB TIP

Refer to "Steps to Enter a New Prescription" (Lab 6), if needed.

Dr. Ramon Ramirez
134 Boylston Street
Cambridge, MA 02139
Office: (617) 479-3400
Fax: (617) 479-3402

Date: _____ 11/21/2017 _____

Patient Name: __ Brian Davidson __

Address: ___ 27 Bradford Street, Newton, MA ___

R_x_ Glucose meter, strip, lancets, solution
Patient choice of meter, noninsulin-
dependent; enough supplies to test tid

Refill: __ 3 __

DEA: AR3587726
State License: 9317432

Dr. R. Ramirez
M.D.

Note: Patient has requested the Breeze 2 meter after reviewing the product in the store. Use the above prescription to complete the following steps:

1. Access the main screen of Visual SuperScript.

2. Click on **FILL Rx's** located on the left side of the menu screen. The *Prescription Processing* form appears.

3. Click on the **NEW Rx** [icon] icon on the top left of the *Prescription Processing* form.

   Note: Prescription information such as the **Rx No.** (prescription number) and **DISPENSE DATE** are automatically generated and added to the form. You may also choose the **Rx ORIGIN** from the drop-down menu if the prescription is not written.

4. Enter your initials in the *Enter Tech Init* box that appears, and click **OK**.

5. Tab to the next data field. This is the **CUSTOMER LOOKUP** text box. Type the first three letters of the customer's last name, and hit **ENTER**.

   Type *DAV* for Brian Davidson as indicated in the sample prescription.

6. Select the appropriate customer by double-clicking on the customer name or by clicking **OK** when the customer name is highlighted in blue.

   Note: The customer's personal information such as **ADDRESS**, **PHONE**, and **BIRTHDATE** will be automatically added to the *Prescription Processing* form.

Note: You are automatically directed to the **Doctor** text box once the patient information is populated. For new prescriptions, the system will search the patient's prescription file to find the name of the prescriber of the most recently filled prescription. If found, then the system will insert the prescriber's name into this field. If a different physician has written the new prescription, then you can delete the old name and enter a new one. For this particular exercise, the physician, Dr. Ramon Ramirez, is listed in the sample prescription and is automatically populated in this field.

7. You will be prompted to the **Prescribed Drug** data entry field. Type in the first three letters of the first prescribed item into the **Prescribed Drug** data entry field. Then press **Enter**.

   Enter *BRE* for the Breeze 2 meter.

8. Select the appropriate drug from the *Drug Name Lookup* dialog box by double-clicking on the drug name or selecting the drug name and clicking **OK**.

9. After receiving approval from the instructor to continue, click **Close** to move through the warnings. Click **Continue Rx** to navigate to the next step.

10. Brand and generic drugs will appear under Available Drug Choices. Use your keyboard's up and down keys to highlight the drug option you want. Press **Enter**. The full drug information appears below, along with an image, if available. Choose the brand name for the drug as specified by the physician—dispense as written (DAW).

11. Next, you will be prompted to the **Refills Ordered** data entry field.

   Key in the appropriate number of refills.

12. Press the **Tab** key. You will be prompted to enter the **Prescribed Quantity**.

   Key in the appropriate quantity in the Prescribed Quantity data entry field.

13. In the **DAW** text box, choose the correct **DAW** code by clicking on the arrow on the right side of the **DAW** data entry field.

   Click on the correct DAW code from the drop-down menu.

Note: When filling a prescription, knowing the correct **DAW** code to be assigned to a prescription is necessary for reimbursement. To accomplish this, distinguish between the brand name and the generic name of the medication. Although the prescriber may write the brand name of a drug on a patient's prescription, it may not necessarily mean that the brand-name drug must be dispensed. If the prescriber indicates **DAW** or "brand name medically necessary" on the patient's prescription for a brand-name drug, then the brand-name drug rather than the generic alternative MUST be dispensed. This situation, for example, would be a **DAW** code 1. Failure to use the proper **DAW** code may result in improper third-party reimbursement to the pharmacy. Seven **DAW** codes are used in the pharmacy practice:

DAW 0—Prescriber has approved the dispensing of a generic medication.
DAW 1—Prescriber requests that the brand-name drug be dispensed.
DAW 2—Prescriber has approved the dispensing of a generic drug, but the patient has requested that the brand-name drug be dispensed.
DAW 3—Pharmacist dispenses the drug as written.
DAW 4—No generic drugs are available in the store.
DAW 5—Brand-name drug is dispensed but is priced as a generic drug.
DAW 6—Registered pharmacist (RPh)–prescriber call is attempted.

14. Press the **Tab** key. Type in the patient abbreviated directions in the **Sig** text box.

   Key in *Use as directed*.

Note: What appears in the blue **Sig in English** space is what will appear on the label. If an error is made when typing in the **Sig**, then backspace to delete the error and retype the correct information.

15. Press the **Tab** key. You will be prompted to enter **Prescribed Days Supply**.

Type in the appropriate days' supply in the **Prescribed Days Supply** data entry field. Enter *30* for the **Prescribed Days Supply**.

 LAB TIP

Most third-party providers will also cover a specific amount of additional supplies, such as gloves or a Sharps container. Medicare, for example, will allow between 100 to 300 lancets and strips every 3 months.

Note: In the **Rx Notes** section, you may add any notes that apply. Because this meter brand was requested by the patient, the **Rx Notes** section is a good place to document it.

Enter *Patient requested the Breeze 2. Technician demonstrated cleaning, use, and testing procedures in store.* Enter the date and your initials.

16. Press the **Enter** key. Click the **Save** icon.

 HINT

Make sure you are saving each prescription using the **Save** button to the right. Use the **Xmit/Record** button once all of the prescriptions are entered to process through insurance.

17. **Continue to add all of the items on the prescription one at a time, and create labels. You will have a total of four items. Each one will need *Use as directed* for its default instructions.**

18. Click on **Label** on the left of the screen to complete adjudication, and **Print** after each item.

19. Prepare the meter and supplies for dispensing, including the label for each product. Affix the second labels to the back of the original prescription.

 LAB TIP

Ask another pharmacy technician student to review your prepared labels for accuracy.

ADDITIONAL EXERCISES

Process the following prescription for Pebbles Flintstone.

 LAB TIP

This prescription is for the inhaler and the spacer.

Note: Prepare the meter and AeroChamber for dispensing, including the label for each product. Affix the second labels to the back of the original prescription.

Dr. Terrance Abbamont
301 Northway
Camillus, NY 13031
Office: (315) 555-4446
Fax: (315) 555-4448

Date: _____8/8/2017_____

Patient Name: ___Pebbles Flintstone___

Address: ___88 Cobblestone Road, Bedrock, NY___

R̽

Proventil 90 mcg MDI
AeroChamber Plus spacer
*patient teaching requested

Refill: ___3___

DEA: BA4477531

_____Dr. T. Abbamont_____
M.D.

Fill the following non-DME supplies for **Cornelia May** *(date of birth [DOB], 11.26.26)*.
- Woun'Dres wound dressing × 1 roll
- Stomahesive Skin Barrier 1¼" × 30 each
- SUR-FIT Natura Drainable Pouch 1¼" (ostomy)

Enter the following non-DME items (Medical nutrition) for **Ronald Gaston** *(DOB 3.22.38)*.
- Ensure Plus nutrition shakes 2 cases (24 cans)
- BD Catheter tip syringes and connectors #35 each

LAB 15

Prescription Verification Using Bar Coding Technology

■ Introduction

A push has been made to automate inventory and dispensing processes for both speed and accuracy. Information systems use a bar coding verification process to ensure the right medication is being dispensed by using the National Drug Code (NDC), lot number, and expiration date.

New systems, such as e-prescribing, eliminate the handwriting interpretation factor, which has accounted for many medication errors in the process. This new system also helps in the inventory and billing processes, because medications are checked in from an order and even counted using automated counters. E-prescribing is still not 100% error free and requires a technician to use the knowledge and skills with which he or she has been trained to review what has been written.

Prescriptions are brought in by hand, electronically sent, or called in from a physician's office. Once a prescription arrives, the preparer can use the bar coding technology to identify the correct medication, based on the printed label. The medication will be either counted by hand or poured into an automated counter machine and prepared for dispensing.

Scanning the bulk bottle verifies the NDC, expiration date, and lot number for the chosen medication. This verification process follows through to the point of sale (POS) systems in most community settings today and ensures that the correct medication is being picked up and charged.

■ Lab Objectives

In this Lab, you will:

- Learn how to verify medications for dispensing by scanning prescriptions and labels using a bar code scanner.
- Prepare medications for dispensing in a community pharmacy, using bar coding technology in the process.

■ Scenario

You are working in a retail pharmacy dispensing area. Your station is the final staging area for **ready** prescriptions. Each prescription must be identified in the **DAILY ACTIVITY LOG** and verified against the bulk medication. The process will consist of scanning the written prescription and recording the NDC in the system. Your instructor will then provide a final check.

■ Pre Lab Information

In previous Lab exercises, you have learned how to print and process labels for retail pharmacy (Labs 1 through 12). You will take the steps learned earlier and add bar coding technology to the process. In addition to verifying the medications needed for each of the prescriptions, you will scan the prescriptions and labels for verification.

■ Student Directions

Estimated completion time: 1 hour

1. Read through the steps in the Lab before performing the Lab exercise.
2. After reading through the Lab, perform the required steps to complete the tasks in each scenario.

1. Access the main screen of Visual SuperScript.

2. Click on **DAILY ACTIVITY LOG** located at the top of the main screen. The *Rx Activity/Batching* dialog box will appear.

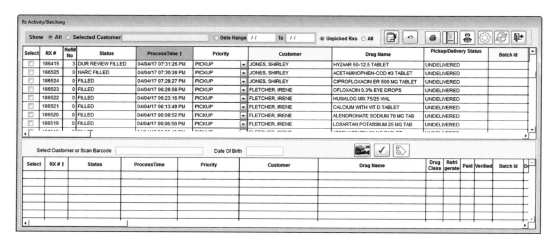

3. Ms. Jones has returned to pick up the prescriptions she dropped off earlier. Place a check mark next to her first prescription in the list, and double-click on her name.

   Note: When you double-click on a customer's name, all of the prescriptions ready to be verified will appear at the bottom of the screen.

4. Click on the **RX VERIFICATION** button.

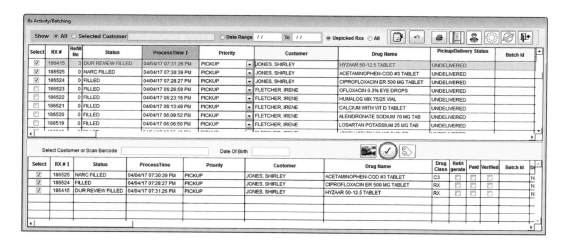

5. The *Final Verification* dialog box will appear. Scan or manually enter the NDC number in the *Enter/Scan NDC* data entry field to ensure the correct bulk medication was used to process the prescription.

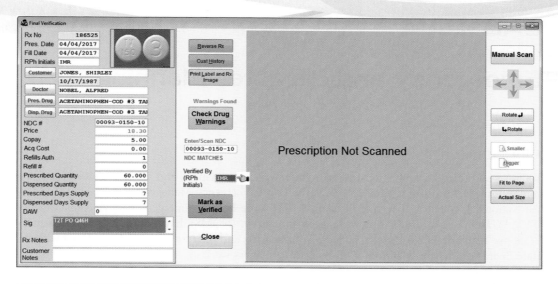

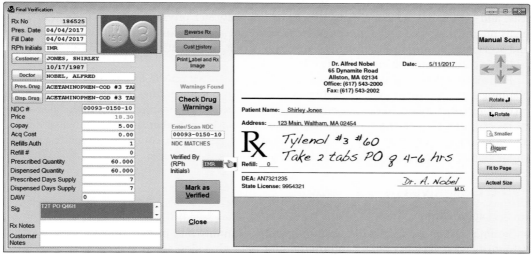

6. Verify the information in the fields found on the left side of the screen. If there are notes or comments needed, they may be entered here as well.

7. Enter your initials into the *Verified By (RPh Initials)* data entry field. Click on the **MARK AS VERIFIED** button and close.

   Note: Final verification must be done by a pharmacist. In this case, your instructor will simulate this review.

8. The *Final Verification* dialog box will continue to appear for each consecutive prescription. Repeat the verification process for each one.

9. Once you have completed verification for each prescription, batch the medications together for patient pickup.

10. Place the batched prescriptions in a pickup area for the instructor to perform final verification.

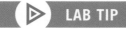 **LAB TIP**

Although you have verified each prescription, the Verified check box will be unmarked in the *Rx Activity/Batching* dialog box until your instructor has performed the final check.

11. Hit the **ESCAPE** button to close.

LAB 16

Emergency and Disaster Planning

■ Introduction

Today's health care workforce must prepare for emergency situations and disasters that impact their community. Government agencies, such as the Local Emergency Management Authority (LEMA), the National Incident Management System (NIMS), the Federal Emergency Management Agency (FEMA), and the National Disaster Management System (NDMS), have set up National Pharmacy Response Teams (NPRTs) that are staffed by pharmacists and pharmacy technicians. Along with the State Boards of Pharmacy and local pharmacies, providers work together to prepare for unexpected events. Pharmacists and pharmacy technicians are vital members of the response team.

Agencies and facilities establish plans that include assignments of tasks and team roles, contact lists, and procedures for handling medications, supplies, and private patient information. These plans require advanced preparation and teamwork to be able to provide patients with medications and services they may need during an emergency event. Special attention is paid to older adults, pediatric patients, and patients who are critically ill.

Pharmacy technicians should demonstrate the ability to participate in emergency and disaster planning for their department or facility, as well as with outside entities. Often stocked or excess medications, such as antibiotics, vaccines, or maintenance medications, are kept in a special inventory. Special delivery procedures may be required, and batteries and other supplies, known as durable and nondurable equipment, may also need to be stocked. All of these components require a process and written plan, including an up-to-date inventory and proper storage.

■ Lab Objectives

In this Lab, you will:

- Be able to demonstrate skills used in disaster planning and preparedness.
- Identify ways to find contact information for patients using electronic profiles.
- Learn the processes to identify and distribute emergency medications, supplies, and equipment needed for patients in the event of a disaster.
- Identify special medications and the procedures required for refrigerated and hazardous medications, as well as those considered waste or requiring disposal.
- Demonstrate ethics, adherence to patient privacy, and team work in a simulated disaster plan or emergency scenario.

ASHP goals 1, 3-9, 11, 13-15, 17-21, 23, 24, 25, 26, 31-35, 37, 38, and 40-44.

■ Scenario

The National Weather Service has issued a hurricane warning for the East coast, and evacuation is mandatory for the three counties in your service area. The long-term care facility you work for currently has 34 patients in house who cannot be evacuated; there are also 12 home-bound patients included under your care. You are also a volunteer of the NPRT, which is responsible for mass vaccines and medications.

■ Pre Lab Information

First, your department's disaster team is responsible for establishing a written plan for responding within 24 hours to provide patients with enough emergency medications, supplies, and equipment to last 7 days. You must make assignments for team members; notify outside staff members, if needed; decide which medications, supplies, and equipment are needed for the list of patients; and plan for inventory control and delivery. Communication is the key; therefore you must also coordinate outside your department and facility with patients, their caregivers, and other organizations.

Estimated completion time: 45 minutes

1. Read through the steps before performing the Lab exercise on your computer.

2. After reading through the Lab, perform the required steps to complete the tasks in each scenario.

3. Answer the questions at the end of the Lab. You should then prepare each medication needed in blister pack 30-day cards for delivery to the Coolidge Nursing Home.

   a. Prepare a written plan (as a group), outlining the following steps:
   - Written policies on how, when, and who will activate the plan
   - Staff assignments, including assignments within your team
   - How notification of staff members will occur
   - How communication with team and media (who and when) will occur
   - How patient privacy and documentation will be kept
   - Ordering and inventory requirements, creating a list of stockpile suggested emergency medications and supplies to keep on hand
   - Creation of a sample policy for delivery and storage recommendations for any special medications, such as insulin and vaccines, as well as refrigerated, high-risk, intravenous (IV), hazardous, over-the-counter (OTC), and controlled medications
   - Examples of basic emergency kit components designed for the diabetic patient

   b. Prepare a *batch* of medications requested for the Coolidge Nursing Home patients to deliver before the hurricane arrives.

   You must first look up the patients in the following list one at a time and find the prescription number for each. Look for the most current prescriptions (dates). You will refill the prescriptions, prepare them using the blister-packing method, and prepare delivery tickets and a billing report for the residents' medications.

   Busch, Jane—Metformin 500 mg
   Busch, John—Lipitor 20 mg and Coumadin
   Ellis, Floyd—Glucolab test strips, lancets, NovoLog, sharps container
   Fletcher, Irene—glipizide, atenolol, and metformin
   Richers, Thelma—Cardizem, hydrochlorothiazide
   Sanchez, Miguel—Plavix 75 mg

STEPS TO PREPARE LABELS FOR A BATCH REFILL

Use the following information to complete the steps listed for each customer.

1. Access the main screen of Visual SuperScript.

2. Click on **FILL Rx's** located on the left side of the menu screen. The *Prescription Processing* form appears.

3. Click on **Cus History/Refill**.

4. Key the first customer name into the **CUSTOMER** data entry field. Press the **ENTER** key. The *Customer Lookup* dialog box appears. Click on the correct customer from the list in the *Customer Lookup* dialog box. Click **OK**.

   Enter customer name *Busch, Jane*.

5. Select the tab titled **PRESCRIPTIONS ON FILE**. Put a checkmark in the checkbox of the first prescription that needs to be refilled.

   Check the box for Metformin 500 mg.

6. Click on **Refill Rx** located at the top of the dialog box.

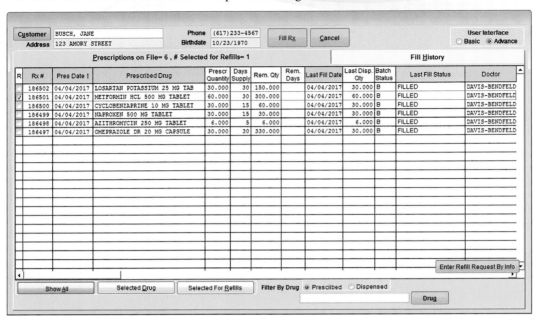

7. The *Prescription Processing* form now returns to the screen. The medication checked in the box will be ready to process. Click on **Xmit/Record** located at the top left of the form, which will prompt the software to adjudication and print a label.

8. Continue with each patient's requested and specific medications by following the previous steps.

STEPS FOR MEDICATION PREPARATION PROCESS

1. Once the labels are printed, retrieve the stock bottles from the shelf for each patient one at a time. Identify the correct medication by verifying the National Drug Code (NDC) number on the bottle and then comparing it with the label.

2. Prepare each blister 30-day card with the individual patient's medications (see Lab 39 for specific instructions). Keep each patient's medications, remaining label or monograph, delivery ticket, and the stock bottle together for verification by the pharmacist.

 LAB TIP

Most pharmacies have a system to ensure completed prescriptions are checked before dispensing, such as using color-coded baskets. Each individual patient has his or her own basket with the ready medications labeled and the stock bottles used for the pharmacist to verify.

STEPS TO PREPARE A BATCH REFILL REPORT

1. Access the main screen of Visual SuperScript.

2. Click on **REPORTS** from the menu toolbar located at the top of the screen.

3. Select **CUSTOMER REPORTS** from the drop-down menu. Then select **CUSTOMER HISTORY** from the expanded menu.

4. A dialog box appears. Notice that the insertion point is in the first data entry field, *Date From*. Type in the date that the *Customer History Report* should start.

> **Type in the date when the batch was filled.**
> **The beginning and ending dates will be the same.**

 LAB TIP

Deleting the default date that appears in the data entry field is not necessary. The date that is keyed in will replace the existing default date.

5. The *Show* field will designate whether the report should be generated to show the copay amount for the medications or the actual price of the medications. Click on the appropriate choice.

> **Select COPAY.**

6. The *Format* field will designate whether the report should be generated in an insurance format or a nursing home (NHome) format.

> **Select NHOME format because the patient is a resident of a nursing home.**

7. Select the *New Page for Each Customer* field if individual pages are desired.

8. The *For* data field offers several choices in generating the *Customer History Report*. Select one of the five choices in which the *Customer History Report* will be generated. Click on the appropriate choice.

> **Select Individual Customer.**

9. The *Customer Name* entry field will ask for the customer name or the name of the insurance plan. The required information depends on the selection made in step 8.

Key in *BUS* for *Busch, Jane.*

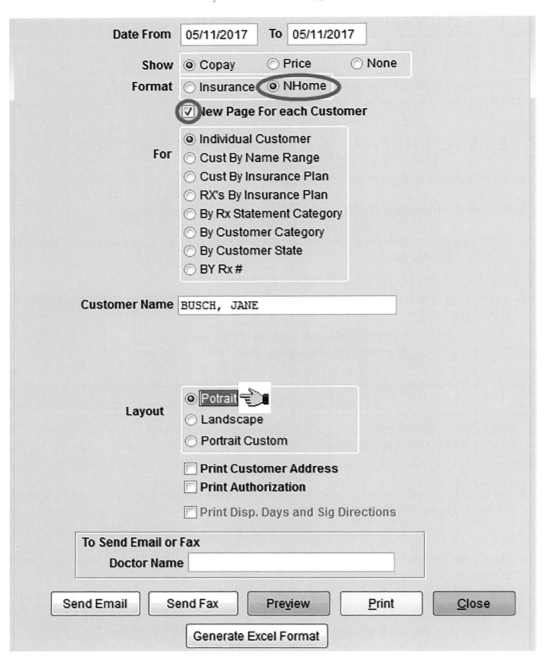

10. Click on **PREVIEW** located at the bottom of the dialog box. The selected *Customer History Report* will open and appear on the screen.

11. Click on the **PRINT REPORT** 🖨 icon located at the top right of the *Report Designer* toolbar.

12. Click on the **CLOSE PREVIEW** ⬛ icon located at the top right of the *Report Designer* toolbar. The report is now closed out, and the dialog box returns.

13. Follow these steps to create a report for each customer on your list. Provide this list, with completed delivery tickets, to the pharmacist for his or her review and verification.

INTERDISCIPLINARY AND TEAM APPROACH CONSIDERATION

Working as a team with other departments will ensure patient deliveries will include everything the patient needs in one run. Other supplies, such as respiratory, feeding, or IV pumps, and OTC items, such as batteries, can be added to the pharmacy supplies (delivery ticket) and medications being sent. Check with other departments before sending a driver, in case there are other needs for the patient.

MEDICATION SAFETY CONSIDERATION

For those medications requiring special storage or refrigeration, include notes on the delivery ticket and in the computer profile for drivers if coolers or ice is required.

HIPAA CONSIDERATION

Anything that is delivered must be recorded on the delivery ticket and signed for by a patient or appropriate caregiver.

RESOURCES

American Diabetes Association, 2015. Retrieved December 21, 2015 from http://www.diabetes.org/living-with-diabetes/treatment-and-care/medication/tips-for-emergency-preparedness.html
ASHP: http://www.ashp.org/DocLibrary/BestPractices/SpecificStEmergPrep.aspx
CDC: Centers for Disease Control Prevention and Control. Retrieved December 21, 2015 from http://emergency.cdc.gov/preparedness/kit/disasters/
FDA: http://www.fda.gov/downloads/EmergencyPreparedness/EmergencyPreparedness/UCM230973.pdf
NABP: http://www.nabp.net/news/assets/06Emergency_Preparedness_Guide.pdf

LAB 17

Medication Therapy Management

■ Introduction

Medication therapy management (MTM) is defined as a broad range of health care services provided by pharmacists and supported by the pharmacy team, especially technicians. As more pharmacy technicians advance their training, attend the American Society of Health-System Pharmacists (ASHP) accredited training programs, and become certified pharmacy technicians, they are becoming invaluable to the management of medication therapy.

As part of a comprehensive patient-care initiative through the Centers for Medicare and Medicaid Services (CMS), the services include medication therapy reviews, pharmacotherapy consults, anti-coagulation management, immunizations, health and wellness programs, and many other clinical services.

For Medicare-eligible patients, specific reporting and other requirements must be met for patients who are receiving services through retail, home health care, and certain other providers.

Many pharmacies are realizing the need to advance the training of pharmacy technicians to support the pharmacist in MTM. With advance training, the pharmacy technician may be able to help with marketing, promoting, scheduling, ordering, record keeping, preparing a report with medication and disease history for the pharmacist from the patient profile, and other duties, depending on specific state laws.

Technicians can assist by preparing the history sections or a *personal medication record (PMR)* from the profile for the pharmacist to review before he or she attends a counseling appointment. In addition, technicians can then perform a *medication therapy review (MTR)*. From this information, the pharmacist can develop a follow-up *medication-related action plan* to help patients get the best benefits from their medications by actively managing drug therapy and by identifying, preventing, and resolving medication-related problems.

MEDICATION SAFETY CONSIDERATION

Remember: Patient profiles are only as complete as you make them. The best practice for creating a complete patient history includes adding notes and over-the-counter (OTC) medications, vitamins, herbals, and durable and nondurable products, such as insulin needles or lancets, to the patient profile. All medications, even those not actually dispensed at your pharmacy, should be included in the profile to ensure that the medication reconciliation report information will be as accurate as possible.

■ Lab Objectives

In this Lab, you will:

- Using the database, look up specific patient profiles and complete the sections of the MTM plan (PMR-written medications and health history) for a pharmacist.
- Prepare a schedule of appointments for the pharmacist to perform MTM counseling.

■ Scenario

You will continue to work together in the simulated laboratory by adding the function of reviewing an electronic health and medication profile and gathering information needed for an MTM for specific patients. These tasks will require performing a search through various fields in the profile, as well as writing legibly and using computer skills, such as preparing reports through Word and Excel.

■ Pre Lab Information

You have learned all the steps of data entry and maintaining a patient profile in a community and institutional setting from previous Labs. Now, you will add the additional practice of reviewing and recording the data found in a profile for a requested patient medication reconciliation report.

■ Student Directions

Estimated completion time: 45 minutes

1. Read through the steps in the Lab before performing the Lab exercise.
2. After reading through the Lab, perform the required steps to create your PMR for the MTM form for a patient.
3. Complete the exercise at the end of the Lab.

STEPS TO REVIEWING A PATIENT'S ELECTRONIC PROFILE AND COMPLETING THE PATIENT'S PERSONAL MEDICATION RECORD

1. Access the main screen of Visual SuperScript.

2. Click on **FILL RX'S** located on the left side of the menu screen. The *Prescription Processing* form appears.

3. Click on the **CUSTOMER'S HISTORY/REFILL** icon on the left of the *Prescription Processing* form, which will provide a complete list of medications for the patient.

4. You will then be prompted to the **CUSTOMER'S LOOKUP** (highlighted in blue) text box. Type the first three letters of the last name, and hit **ENTER**.

   Type *SAN* for Sanchez, Miguel. Validate the date of birth (DOB): 7.21.1954

5. Select the appropriate customer by double-clicking on the customer name or by clicking **OK**. The customer's profile with all medications that have been entered into the database will be listed.

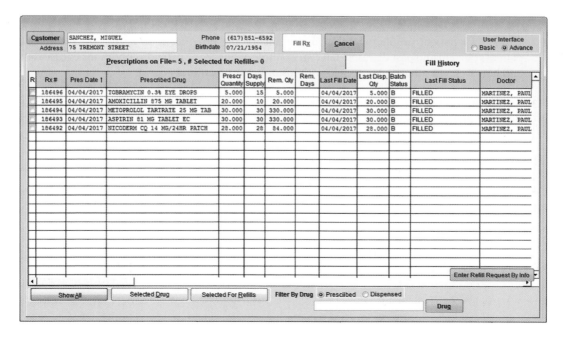

LAB TIP

Remember: In the outpatient setting, pharmacy technicians are often the first member of the pharmacy team to receive the prescription. A trained pharmacy technician can review the prescription for potential errors and alert the pharmacist, enabling the pharmacist to interview the patient or call the physician as needed.

6. Use the **PRNT SCRN** function to share this with your partner and instructor for review.

7. Using the form provided in Lab 49, complete the sections of the MTM form with the medication history, and ask your partner to check this against your **PRNT SCRN** document.

8. Click **CANCEL**, and then close the *Prescription Processing* dialog box.

9. Click on the **CUSTOMERS** icon on the left, and look up the patient history screen.

    Enter *SAN* for Sanchez, Miguel.

10. Beginning with the demographics (address, phone, birth date, and other personal information) and payment information, fill out the MTM form in these areas.

11. Then click on each tab at the bottom, starting with allergies. Review this section by clicking on the various tabs, record information for allergies; diseases; diet; laboratory, ancillary, and rehabilitation orders; or any other required information to complete the form.

12. Together with the **PRNT SCRN** from the **CUSTOMER HISTORY/REFILL** tab, ask a fellow student to review the MTM form after your areas have been completed.

13. Once completed, provide the printed screen and the MTM form for a final check by the instructor (pharmacist).

REVIEW QUESTIONS

1. Why is it important to include herbals and vitamins in a patient's profile? Give an example of an interaction.

2. Using your patient profile, why is it important for the pharmacist to know and record the patient's current and past diseases? Give an example of one of the patient's conditions or diseases, and how wellness education can help with his or her medications.

3. As a technician, what role can you play in the MTM process in your state? (Use your State Board of Pharmacy Web site and working technicians as a reference.)

RESOURCE

Centers for Medicare & Medicaid Services, *Medication Therapy Management*. Retrieved August 18, 2014, from http://www.cms.gov/Medicare/Prescription-Drug-Coverage/PrescriptionDrugCovContra/MTM.html

LAB 18

Special Medications—Risk Evaluation and Mitigation Strategies (iPledge) Program

■ Introduction

Special medications require additional documentation that follows prescribing guidelines similar to those followed for Schedule II (CII) controlled substances. The U.S. Food and Drug Administration (FDA) regulates certain drugs because of the increased risks of birth defects and other severe adverse effects through a program known as ***Risk Evaluation and Mitigation Strategies (REMS)***. Accutane or isotretinion, used for severe acne, requires the physician, pharmacist, and all female patients to register with the ***iPledge*** program, consent to treatment, and understand the risks of becoming pregnant. Male patients must also sign consent to treatment by acknowledging the increased risks of adverse effects.

Knowing the requirements for special medications is a must for pharmacy technicians who will be responsible for following the guidelines.

MEDICATION SAFETY CONSIDERATION

If you are unsure whether a medication is considered an **REMS** or **iPledge** medication, then use the FDA Web site to search for it at www.fda.gov.

■ Lab Objectives

In this Lab, you will:

- Identify whether a special medication is an investigational drug or under the REMS program and use the necessary resources to follow any special considerations that are required.
- Demonstrate the steps required to interpret a prescription for a special medication, using software data entry skills in a simulated laboratory environment.
- Verify each other's work (simulate tech-check-tech [TCT]) when performing data entry and prescription data entry.

ASHP goals: 3, 8, 12, 17, 18, 35, 36, and 41.

■ Scenario

Today, you are working in a simulated retail setting and processing medications considered *special* as either investigational or included in the FDA's **REMS** (**iPledge**) program.

■ Pre Lab Information

The Lab exercise will teach you how to identify, document, and perform the steps for dispensing a special medication such as an investigational drug or a medication under the REMS iPledge program.

LAB TIP

Review the iPledge program at https://www.ipledgeprogram.com/ before beginning.

Estimated completion time: 30 minutes

1. Read through the steps in the Lab before performing the Lab exercise.
2. After reading through the Lab, perform the required steps to enter provider information.
3. Complete the exercise at the end of the Lab.

STEPS TO PROCESSING A PRESCRIPTION FOR AN iPLEDGE MEDICATION

Dr. Ramon Ramirez
134 Boylston Street
Cambridge, MA 02139
Office: (617) 479-3400
Fax: (617) 479-3402

Date: ___11/21/2017___

Patient Name: ___Marjorie Davidson___

Address: ___27 Bradford Street, Newton, MA___

Rx

Claravis 30 mg
Sig: 1 tab bid

Refill: ___0___

DEA: AR3587726
State License: 9317432

Dr. R. Ramirez
M.D.

1. Process the above prescription.

Note: Keep in mind that this medication is available only as a prepackaged unit that cannot be broken. The medication is dispensed as a 90-day fill for 227 units and a 114-day supply. These fields will be prepopulated.

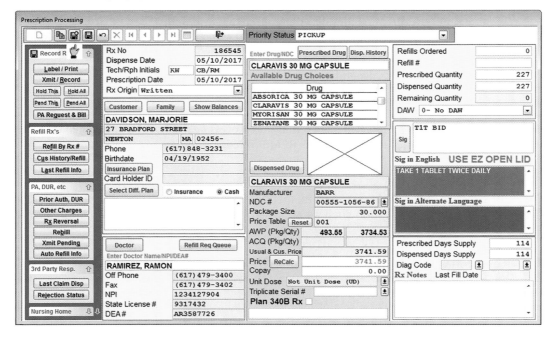

2. Prepare the medication for dispensing, including labeling the product. Affix the second label to the back of the original prescription.

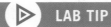

LAB TIP

Ask another pharmacy technician student to review your prepared label for accuracy.

3. Visit the Web site https://www.ipledgeprogram.com/ to answer the following questions.

4. Use the iPledge Program Patient Introductory Brochure, and name three steps the patient must follow to dispense isotretinion (Accutane).

5. Female patients do not have to meet the birth control requirements if they meet certain qualifications. Name three of these.

6. Name two steps that female patients must take each month before getting a new prescription.

LAB 19

Investigational Drugs and Tobacco Products

■ Introduction

An investigational drug is a medication that is still under study and does not yet have approval from the U.S. Food and Drug Administration (FDA) to be legally marketed and sold in the United States. As new products, such as smokeless tobacco, are introduced, the FDA must review the safety and health concerns to the public and consider regulations to include warnings, an over-the-counter (OTC) versus a prescription medication, and even advertising.

FDA approval is the final step in the process of drug development. The first step in the process is for the new drug to be tested in the laboratory. If the results are promising, then the drug company or sponsor must apply for FDA approval to test the drug in people through an Investigational New Drug (IND) application. Once the IND application is approved, clinical trials can begin. Clinical trials are research studies conducted to determine the safety and measure the effectiveness of the drug in people. Once clinical trials are completed, the drug company or sponsor submits the study results in a New Drug Application (NDA) or a Biologics License Application (BLA) to the FDA. This application is carefully reviewed and, if the drug is found to be reasonably safe and effective, it is approved. Most common, investigational drugs include those associated with:

- Cancers
- Human immunodeficiency virus (HIV)
- Autoimmune diseases (e.g., rheumatoid arthritis)
- Myocardial infarctions (i.e., heart attacks)

The most common way that a patient can be given an IND is by *participating in a clinical trial* sponsored by the drug company. A patient's physician may suggest participation in a clinical trial as one treatment option, or a patient or family member can ask a physician about clinical trials or INDs available to treat cancer, for example.

Physicians are required to follow strict guidelines, including gaining approval from their Institutional Review Board and obtaining informed consent from the patient. Informed consent is a process that includes a document to be signed by the patient, which outlines the known risks and benefits of the treatment, as well as the rights and responsibilities of the patient.

Pharmacy technicians play an important role in the documentation, inventory, and preparation of these drugs in a hospital setting. When preparing an intravenous (IV) IND, technicians will be asked to keep special documentation separately, as well as an inventory in a secured area in the pharmacy away from FDA-approved drugs. In most cases, any remaining amounts of the drug and all containers are usually sent back to the manufacturer after the trial is complete.

■ Lab Objectives

In this Lab, you will:

- Research some current investigational drugs, and use available resources to follow any special considerations that are required.
- Demonstrate the steps required to prepare an informed consent, receive an investigational drug, and interpret a prescription using software data entry skills in a simulated laboratory environment.
- Review a sample standard operating procedure (SOP) for investigational drugs.
- Review smokeless tobacco products and FDA guidelines.

ASHP goals: 3, 8, 11, 14, 16, 17, 19, 21, 23, 24, 25, 33, 35, 41, 42, 43, and 45.

▪ Scenario

Today, you are working in a simulated hospital retail setting with specific documentation and medications that are considered *investigational*.

▪ Pre Lab Information

The Lab exercise will teach you how to identify an investigational drug, to process the necessary documentation, and to perform the steps for dispensing and receiving the investigational drug in the inventory.

▪ Student Directions

Estimated completion time: 30 minutes

1. Read through the steps in the Lab before performing the Lab exercise.
2. After reading through the Lab, perform the required steps to complete the informed consent.
3. Complete the exercise at the end of the Lab.

STEPS FOR PROCESSING A PRESCRIPTION FOR AN INVESTIGATIONAL MEDICATION

Dr. Richard Kaplan
5906 North Mahagony Street
Marshfield, MA 02050
Refills: (781) 555-7303
Fax: (781) 555-7302

Date: _____12/2/2017_____

Patient Name: __Patrisha Divine_____

Address: ___77823 Ferry Street, Marshfield, MA 02050_____

℞ *Actemra 8 mg/kg IV q 4 wks*
Brand necessary

Refill: __0__

DEA: BK1234424

Dr. R. Kaplan
M.D.

---

1. Process the above prescription.

 LAB TIP

The patient's weight is 103 pounds. You must convert pounds to kilograms and determine how many milligrams must be dispensed.

2. Prepare the medication for dispensing, including labeling the product. Affix the second label to the back of the original prescription.

 LAB TIP

Ask another pharmacy technician student to review your prepared label for accuracy.

1. Visit the Web site from the National Cancer Institute (http://www.cancer.gov/about-cancer/treatment/clinical-trials/search), find an investigational drug of choice, and complete the informed consent documentation form on Evolve.

2. Perform an Internet search to respond to the following questions or statements:

   A. What acronyms apply to tobacco products that the FDA regulates?

   B. Name two risks that are posted on the FDA Web site for these products.

   C. Name four warnings that are required for smokeless tobacco products per the Family Smoking Prevention and Tobacco Control Act.

   D. This warning content must cover at least how much of the printed advertisement?

LAB 20

Reconstitution and Flavoring Pediatric Medications

▪ Introduction

Patient noncompliance with taking prescribed medication costs billions of dollars each year and can lead to excessive hospital visits and even death. Pediatric medications are especially difficult for parents to give because of poor taste, especially in liquid doses.

Flavoring medications is a way to promote compliance, not only in humans but in animals as well. Flavor choices can be sweet to semisweet and chocolate or even beef, liver, chicken, and other delicious flavors for animals. Most pediatric medications come as powders, which must be reconstituted (have liquid added to them) at the time of dispensing. They may be salty, sour, or bitter, and may need to have flavoring added at the time of reconstitution.

Not every medication can be flavored with any flavor. The amount of water to add is written on the medication bottle, and the correct flavoring agent combination is provided by the manufacturer or other agent. Flavoring could be drops of one flavor or a combination of several. The pharmacy technicians must learn to follow directions, similar to baking a cake, and properly perform this function. In addition, technicians must communicate proper storage and dispensing instructions to the patients or parents.

▪ Lab Objectives

In this Lab, you will:

- Demonstrate the skills required for reconstituting and flavoring a pediatric medication.
- Prepare an electronic label from a prescription for a pediatric liquid medication.
- Use a written recipe to flavor a pediatric medication.
- Identify special requirements for reconstituted medications including auxiliary labels and patient directions for storage.
- Demonstrate ethics, adhere to patient privacy, and work with team members in a simulated laboratory scenario.

▪ Scenario

In your pharmacy today, you have several patients who have brought in prescriptions for pediatric suspensions that must be filled. Once a label is prepared, you must reconstitute and flavor each one according to the directions provided in this Lab exercise. The final products must have proper labeling, include an oral dose spoon in the bag, be checked by your instructor (simulating the pharmacist verification process), dispensed, and charged for using a cash register.

▪ Pre Lab Information

Using the Visual Superscript database and the prescriptions, medications, and supplies provided, review the process for flavoring and reconstitution of your prescriptions. Use a reference source to find storage information and to identify any auxiliary labels required before entering prescription.

▪ Student Directions

Estimated completion time: 1.5 hours

1. Read through the steps before performing the Lab exercise on your computer.
2. After reading through the Lab, perform the required steps to complete the tasks in each scenario.
3. Answer the questions at the end of the Lab.

Dr. Ramon Ramirez
134 Boylston Street
Cambridge, MA 02139
Office: (617) 479-3400
Fax: (617) 479-3402

Date: _7/15/2017_

Patient Name: __Benjamin Dawson__

Address: __7755 Walnut Street, Newton, MA__

℞

Tamiflu susp. 12 mg/mL
45 mg bid x 5 days
Discard any remaining amount

Refill: __0__

DEA: AR3587726

Dr. R. Ramirez
M.D.

---

1. Process the above prescription.

2. The physician has ordered 45 mg twice a day, and 12 mg are in every milliliter of medication. To calculate the amount needed to dispense, use the following directions. First, determine how many milliliters and teaspoons the patient will need to take in one dose.

$$\frac{12 \text{ mg}}{1 \text{ mL}} = \frac{45 \text{ mg}}{x} = 3.75 \text{ mL (to be taken twice a day} = 7 \text{ mL)}$$

Next, convert the 3.75 mL to teaspoons (conversion is 5 mL = 1 teaspoon)

$$\frac{3.75 \text{ mL}}{x} = \frac{5 \text{ mL}}{\text{tsp}} = 0.75 \text{ or } ¾ \text{ tsp (a total of 1.5 tsp daily} \times 5 \text{ days)}$$

Type in *Take ¾ teaspoon (3.75 mL) twice daily for 5 days. Discard the remaining.*

MEDICATION SAFETY CONSIDERATION

When typing directions for pediatric medications, use the best practice of typing the amount of the dose in milliliters, not only teaspoons or tablespoons. For example: Type "Give 1 teaspoon (5 mL) three times a day." Household utensils can vary from 2.5 to 17 mL in some cases.

Note: When dispensing pediatric oral suspensions, full bottles must be dispensed. This order will require a total of 37.5 mL for the 5 days (7 mL × 5 days). You will need to prepare and enter a charge for two bottles (50 mL) total in the prescribed quantity field.

3. Prepare the medication for dispensing, including labeling the product. Affix the second label to the back of the original prescription. Affix any auxiliary labels that apply.

4. Once the labels are printed, retrieve the stock bottles from the shelf for each patient one at a time. Identify the correct medication by verifying the NDC number on the bottle compared with the printed label.

LAB TIP

Each medication has a specific NDC number provided by the U.S. Food and Drug Administration (FDA). To verify that the correct medication is being used for each prescription, this number must match the stock bottle from the shelf to the prescription printed.

EXERCISE

1. Prepare each medication by following the directions on the label for amount of water to add.

    See each prescription at the end of the Lab.

2. Follow the procedure for flavoring each medication.

    Amoxil—Flavor each bottle using a bubblegum agent; add 0.9 mL to reconstituted bottle, and gently shake.

    Tamiflu—Flavor each bottle using a flavoring agent, add 0.3 mL grape and 0.2 mL bubblegum to reconstituted bottle, and gently shake.

    Augmentin—Flavor each bottle using 0.6 mL grape and 1.1 mL of bubblegum agents. Gently shake.

    Cephalexin—Flavor each bottle using 1.1 mL of orange flavoring agent.

    Zithromax—Flavor using either 0.3 mL of orange flavoring agent OR 0.2 mL grape and 0.3 mL bubblegum (per customer preference).

3. Label each bottle, and add any auxiliary labels required (based on the reference information found).

4. Include an oral dose spoon or syringe for the patient. Keep each patient's medications and remaining label and monograph, flavoring agent, and syringe or dropper together for pharmacist verification.

 LAB TIP

Keep the syringe or dropper, the flavoring agent bottle that was used to measure, and the recipe and directions as part of the pharmacist verification process.

5. Once the pharmacist has completed the verification process, simulate the dispensing to include customer interaction, processing the sale, and final packaging.

INTERDISCIPLINARY AND TEAM APPROACH CONSIDERATION

Communication is especially important when filling a sick child's medication. Often the parents are distracted and will not really look at the medication until they get home. Writing or typing the instructions on the label is best and will help ensure better compliance when parents and other caregivers, such as grandparents, are home. Taking the extra few minutes to explain the directions or to offer the pharmacist's time for questions is worth it.

MEDICATION SAFETY CONSIDERATION

For those medications requiring special storage or refrigeration, use auxiliary labels if required. These labels are colored and designed to be eye catching.

Using an oral dose syringe or spoon will ensure that the parent always gives the correct dose in milliliters. It is very easy to make a mistake when using the common teaspoon and tablespoon for correct doses once the parents or caregivers are at home. Household utensils can vary from 2.5 to 17 mL in some cases.

Community Pharmacy Practice

Be sure to verify that a patient profile authorization for health information for minors is in the system when dispensing children's medications.

Dr. Ronald Zimmerman
609 Spruce Street
Chestnut Hill, MA 02167
Office: (617) 556-7200
Fax: (617) 556-7202

Date: ___6/6/2017___

Patient Name: ___Teressa Powers___

Address: ___4237 West Willow Street, Westwood, MA___

R_x

Amoxil 125 mg/mL susp.
3/4 tsp bid x 10 days
Discard any remaining amount.

Refill: ___0___

DEA: AZ2532118

Dr. R. Zimmerman
M.D.

Dr. Ramon Ramirez
134 Boylston Street
Cambridge, MA 02139
Office: (617) 479-3400
Fax: (617) 479-3402

Date: ___10/21/2017___

Patient Name: ___Jason Moran___

Address: ___5534 West Ash Street, Gloucester, MA___

R_x

Augmentin 400 mg/5 mL susp.
1½ tsp q 12 hours x 10 days

Refill: ___0___ Discard any remaining amount

DEA: AR3587726

Dr. R. Ramirez
M.D.

Dr. Ramon Ramirez
134 Boylston Street
Cambridge, MA 02139
Office: (617) 479-3400
Fax: (617) 479-3402

Date: _12/31/2017_

Patient Name: _Larry Jones_

Address: _100 King Street, Boston, MA_

R̽x

Cephalexin 500 mg/5 mL susp.
2 tsp q 12 hours x 7 days

Refill: _0_   *Discard any remaining amount*

DEA: AR3587726

Dr. R. Ramirez
M.D.

Dr. Terrance Abbomont
300 Stainford Street
Springfield, MA 01104
Office: (413) 776-9000
Fax: (413) 776-9001

Date: _8/22/2017_

Patient Name: _Adel Wilson_

Address: _5090 West Willow Street, Westwood, MA_

R̽x

Zithromax 200 mg/5 mL susp.
400 mg x 1 day, then ¾ tsp x 4 days

Refill: _0_

DEA: BA4477531

Dr. T. Abbomont
M.D.

RESOURCE

Mosby's Drug Reference for Health Professions, ed 4, St Louis, 2014, Mosby.

LAB 21

Entering Immunization Syringes (Batch Preparation)

■ Introduction

Community and institutional pharmacies offer immunizations to patients as part of well care or preventative treatment. The medication is supplied in **minivials** that are 1- or 2-mL container vials and can be a solution or powder that must be diluted.

Often, the pharmacy will prepare the doses ahead of time and refrigerate them in anticipation of a special day or time of year when patients frequently come in. These syringes should be prepared using aseptic technique and must be appropriately labeled for the pharmacist to use.

■ Lab Objectives

In this Lab, you will:

- Interpret and calculate an immunization (intravenous [IV]) order.
- Prepare labels and syringes for simulated measles, mumps, and rubella injections.

■ Pre Lab Information

A pharmacy technician may be instructed to prepare several syringes with specific doses for immunizations ahead of a clinic or community event. Each medication must be checked using the National Drug Code (NDC) number, lot number, and verification of the manufacturer's expiration date. Labels can be prepared ahead of time for each syringe. You will prepare a batch of 10 syringes of simulated measles, mumps, and rubella virus live 0.5 mL/dose vaccines for your facility. They will require individual labeling, refrigeration, an auxiliary label, and be given a beyond-use date (the Lab will provide instructions).

■ Student Directions

Estimated completion time: 60 minutes

1. Read through the steps in the Lab before performing the Lab exercise.
2. After reading through the Lab, perform the required steps to enter compounded drug information.
3. Practice entering a new drug and preparing labels for syringes for immunization administration.
4. Prepare 10 syringes of simulated measles, mumps, and rubella virus live 0.5 mL/dose vaccines.

STEPS TO ENTER THE NEW MEASLES, MUMPS, AND RUBELLA SYRINGE (DRUG)

1. Access the main screen of Visual SuperScript.

2. Select **Drugs** from the drop-down menu. A dialog box entitled *Drugs* will pop up.

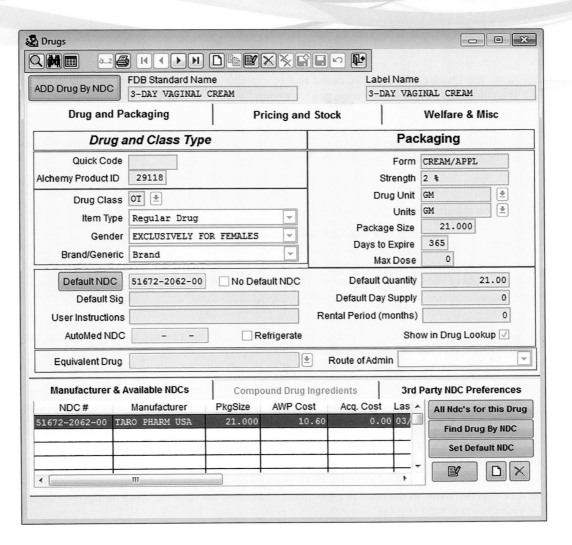

3. Click on the **NEW** [icon] icon located on the toolbar at the top of the *Drugs* dialog box. The form is now ready for you to enter information about the compounded drug.

4. Click on the *Label Name* data entry field.

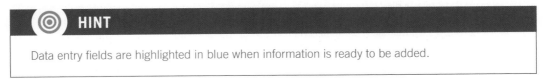

HINT

Data entry fields are highlighted in blue when information is ready to be added.

5. Type in the name of the compounded order that will appear on the label.

Enter *MMR syringe*.

Note: Three tabbed pages are provided on this form: (1) **DRUG AND PACKAGING**; (2) **PRICING AND STOCK**; and (3) **WELFARE & MISC**.

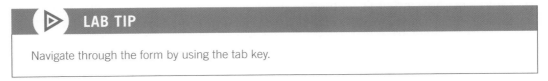

LAB TIP

Navigate through the form by using the tab key.

6. Type the following into the *Quick Code* data entry field:

Enter MMRSYR.

Note: The *Quick Codes* field is a useful tool to expedite the search for drugs in your database. The codes that you enter for your new compound should be based on the label name of the compound.

7. Click on the arrow to the right of the *Drug Class* field. The *Drug Class* dialog box appears. Click on the appropriate drug class from the drop-down list. Click **OK**.

Select Rx.

8. Click on the arrow to the right of *Item Type*. A list of drug items appears.

Click on Compound from this list.

9. Indicate whether the new compound is gender-specific in the *Gender* field. Click on the arrow to the right of the *Gender* field to access the drop-down list.

Select Both.

10. Tab to the *Brand/Generic* field. Click on the arrow to the right of the field. Identify the new compound as brand or generic by clicking on the appropriate choice.

Select Generic.

11. Click on the arrow to the right of the *Drug Unit* field. The *Dispensing Unit* dialog box appears. Click on the appropriate dispensing unit from the list. Click **OK**.

Select ML.

Note: *EA* means *each*; *GM* means *gram*; *ML* means *milliliter*.

12. Click on the arrow to the right of *Units*. The *Units* dialog box appears. Click on the appropriate unit from this list. Click **OK**.

Select ML.

13. Tab to the *Package Size* field.

Enter 0.5 (for 0.5 mL) for the package size.

MEDICATION SAFETY CONSIDERATION

For this exercise, we will use a simulated measles, mumps, and rubella vaccine that has been reconstitued with diluent; it must be used within 8 hours and refrigerated.

Each vaccine will have information and specific manufacturer recommendation regarding storage. For this drug, use the shortest time allowed in the program for now.

14. Tab to *Days to Expire*.

Enter 1 day.

15. Click on the *Default Sig* field. Because the manufacturer recommends storage after dilution and to use it within 8 hours, we will add the following message in the default field.

Enter Use as directed within 8 hrs.

16. Click on the **SAVE** 💾 icon located at the top right of the toolbar. Basic information regarding the new compound has now been saved to the *Drugs* form.

17. You are now ready to add the ingredient(s) of the new compound to the *Drugs* form. The bottom section of the *Drugs* form has three tabbed pages: (1) **Manufacturing & Available NDCs**; (2) **Compound Drug Ingredients**; and (3) **3rd Party NDC Preferences**.

Click on Compound Drug Ingredients.

18. Each additive and amount needed in the new compound will be added one at a time to the grid. Click on the **New** 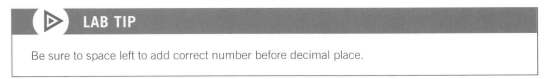 icon located at the bottom right of this *Drugs* form. Two dialog boxes pop up on the screen: *Drug Name Lookup* and *Compound Drug Ingredients*.

19. Key in the first few letters of the desired drug ingredient. Select the correct drug from the list by clicking on the drug name. Click **OK**.

Enter MMR for measles, mumps, and rubella virus vaccine live 0.5 mL/dose.

20. Enter the quantity needed for the MMR vial.

Enter 0.5 (for 0.5 mL).

> ▷ **LAB TIP**
>
> Be sure to space left to add correct number before decimal place.

21. Click on the **Save** button on the bottom of the *Compound Drug Ingredients* dialog box.

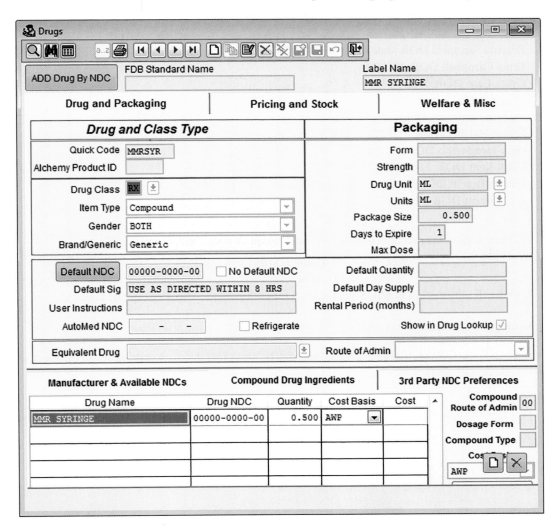

22. Click on the **CLOSE** ⏻ icon located at the top right of the toolbar. You have completed the task of adding a new vaccine order to the pharmacy computer system!

23. You are now returned to the main screen. Perform a drug look-up procedure to ensure that the new compound has been correctly added to the computer system.

    a. Select the **DRUG** button.

    b. Click on the **FIND** 🔍 icon located at the top left of the toolbar.

    c. The *Drug Name Lookup* dialog box appears. Type in the label name of the new compound.
        Enter *MMR* for measles, mumps, and rubella to search for syringes 0.5 mL,
                or use the QUICK CODE you selected—*MMRSYR*

    d. Select the correct compound from the list by clicking on the drug name. Click **OK**.

    e. Read through the *Drugs* form to check for accuracy. Click the **COMPOUND DRUG INGREDI-ENTS** tab at the bottom of the screen to verify ingredients.

    f. Click on the **CLOSE** ⏻ icon on the top right of the toolbar to clear the screen.

STEPS TO CREATE PATIENT LABELS (10) FOR THE MEASLES, MUMPS, AND RUBELLA (MMR) SYRINGES

Using the steps in the prescription entry process (Lab 6), enter the IV order for each of the patients who will be getting the vaccine during the clinic today.

List of patients:

Evarista Sandoval DOB (date of birth): 1/18/74
Erma Campbell DOB: 10/3/24
Grace Cato DOB: 7/30/14
Maureen Finnegan DOB: 1/6/56
Pebbles Flintstone DOB: 1/1/73
Ernest Hatcher DOB: 3/28/29
Gary Henderson DOB: 4/30/47
Clark Kent DOB: 11/15/46
Brenda Leavitt DOB: 2/20/46
Paul Leavitt DOB: 12/25/48

1. When adding the prescribed drug, use the drug quick code created for the syringe.

    Enter *MMRSYR*.

2. Once all information is added, print a label for each patient. Affix a refrigerate label.

3. Aseptically prepare the syringes.

4. Prepare the syringes for the instructor to check by providing the stock vials used and the finished syringes (labeled).

Nonsterile Compounding

LAB 22

Extemporaneous Compounding

■ Introduction

Extemporaneous, or nonsterile, compounding is a common function of pharmacy practice. This process of preparing dosages or forms of medications may not be available from the manufacturer or may not be appropriate for the patient. For example, pediatric and geriatric patients may require a form that can be more easily swallowed.

Dosage forms can include ointments, creams, lotions, suppositories, gels, capsules, tablets, and even lozenges and lollipops. Extemporaneous compounding is similar to baking in that special instructions and the order of mixing should be considered, as well as the required calculations.

Technicians must use math, reading, and pharmacology skills and understand the procedures and equipment that will be used to compound. Special guidelines, known as Good Manufacturing Practices (GMPs), are established by the U.S. Food and Drug Administration (FDA) and are designed to provide safe and effective products for customers. In addition, USP Chapter 795 provides specific instructions for labeling, processing, facilities and equipment, and training of personnel in this role.

■ Lab Objectives

In this Lab, you will:

- Enter new compounded drug data in the pharmacy software database.

■ Pre Lab Information

A patient will often require a specific dose or dose form that is not available from the manufacturer. A physician may order a special "compound" to be made by the pharmacy, which will be presented as a prescription. The following exercise demonstrates how to enter a compound prescription in the database and allows or charges all of the ingredients. Once completed, you will be able to process a compound prescription for a specific patient through a *Quick Challenge*.

■ Student Directions

Estimated completion time: 30 minutes

1. Read through the steps in the Lab before performing the Lab exercise.
2. After reading through the Lab, perform the required steps to enter the compounded drug information.
3. Practice filling a prescription using the new compounded drug information.

STEPS TO ENTER COMPOUND DRUG INFORMATION

1. Access the main screen of Visual SuperScript.

2. Select **DRUGS** from the drop-down menu. A dialog box entitled *Drugs* will pop up.

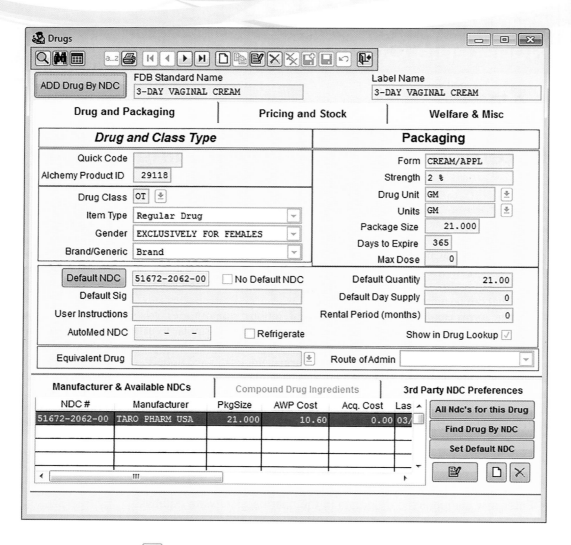

3. Click on the **NEW** ⬜ icon located on the toolbar at the top of the *Drugs* dialog box. The form is now ready for you to enter information concerning the compounded drug.

4. Click on the *Label Name* data entry field.

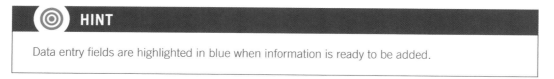

HINT

Data entry fields are highlighted in blue when information is ready to be added.

5. Type in the name of the compounded drug that will appear on the vial label.

Enter *Anna's Antiwrinkle Cream.*

Note: Three tabbed pages appear in this form: (1) **DRUG AND PACKAGING**; (2) **PRICING AND STOCK**; and (3) **WELFARE & MISC**.

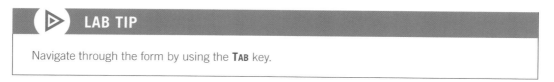

LAB TIP

Navigate through the form by using the **TAB** key.

6. Type the following into the *Quick Code* data entry field:

Enter *Annaaw.*

Note: The *Quick Code* field is a useful tool to expedite the search for drugs in your database. The codes that you enter for your new compound should be based on the label name of the compound.

7. Key in the *Alchemy Product ID* for the new compounded drug.

Enter *MD2017*
for Marjorie Davidson, year 2017, on the master FR.

 LAB TIP

The *Alchemy Product ID* is the lot number that was created by the pharmacy for the new compounded drug. This lot number or *Alchemy Product ID* must be six characters or less.

8. Click on the arrow to the right of the *Drug Class* field. The *Drug Class* dialog box appears. Click on the appropriate drug class from the drop-down list. Click **OK**.

Select Rx.

9. Click on the arrow to the right of *Item Type*. A list of drug items appears.

Click on Compound from this list.

10. Indicate whether the new compound is gender-specific in the *Gender* field. Click on the arrow to the right of the *Gender* field to access the drop-down list.

Select Both.

11. Tab to the *Brand/Generic* field. Click on the arrow to the right of the field. Identify the new compound as brand- or generic-specific by clicking on the appropriate choice.

Select Generic.

12. Click on **DEFAULT SIG**. This new compound may be frequently prescribed with the same instructions for use. Enter the appropriate instructions for use in the text field. If needed, these default instructions may be changed when filling the prescription.

Enter *Apply to affected area.*

13. Click on the *Drug Unit* field on the right side of the *Drug and Packaging* form.

14. Click on the arrow to the right of *Drug Unit* field. The *Dispensing Unit* dialog box appears. Click on the appropriate dispensing unit from the list. Click **OK**.

Select GM.

Note: *EA* means *each*; *GM* means *gram*; *ML* means *milliliter.*

15. Click on the arrow to the right of *Units*. The *Units* dialog box appears. Click on the appropriate unit from this list. Click **OK**.

Select GM.

16. Click on the **Save** 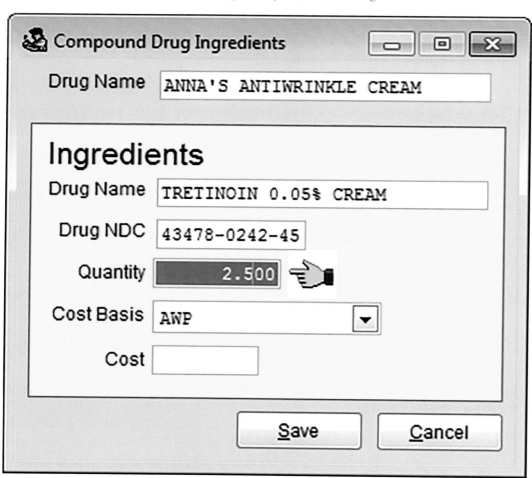 icon located at the top right of the toolbar. Basic information regarding the new compound has been saved to the *Drugs* form. You are now ready to add the ingredients of the new compound to the *Drugs* form. The bottom section of the *Drugs* form has three tabbed pages: (1) **Manufacturing & Available NDCs**; (2) **Compound Drug Ingredients**; and (3) **3rd Party NDC Preferences**.

    Note: *NDC* means *National Drug Code*.

    Click on **Compound Drug Ingredients**.

17. Each ingredient in the new compound will be added one at a time to the grid. Click on the **New** icon located at the bottom right of this *Drugs* form. Two dialog boxes will appear on the screen: *Drug Name Lookup* and *Compound Drug Ingredients*.

18. Key in the first few letters of the desired drug ingredient. Select the correct drug from the list by clicking on the drug name. Click **OK**.

    Enter *Tret* for Tretinoin 0.05% Cream.
    Select the 45.0 package size for this drug.

19. Highlight the correct medication needed, based on your prescription.

20. In the *Compound Drug Ingredients* dialog box, type in the correct quantity of drug (in grams) that you will need.

    For this compound, you will need 2.5 g.

Compound Drug Ingredients

Drug Name ANNA'S ANTIWRINKLE CREAM

Ingredients

Drug Name TRETINOIN 0.05% CREAM

Drug NDC 43478-0242-45

Quantity 2.500

Cost Basis AWP

Cost

Save   Cancel

21. Click the **Save** icon on the bottom of the *Compound Drug Ingredients* dialog box.

22. Continue to add each ingredient one at a time by clicking on the **New** 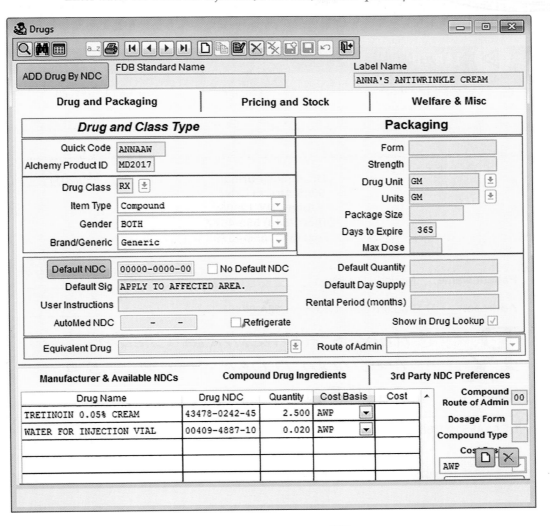 icon located at the bottom right of the *Drugs* form. Review steps 18 through 21 to add each ingredient.

Enter *water* for water for injection, 5 mL vial, and the quantity of *0.02 mL*.

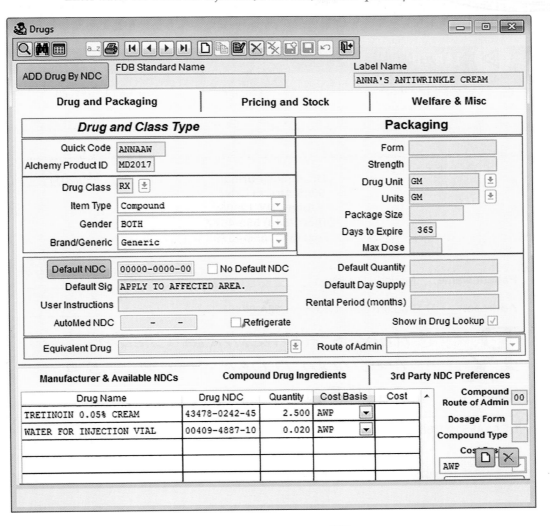

23. Once all of the ingredients are added, click the **Close** 🔳 icon on the top right of the dialog box. The compound is now saved.

24. You are now returned to the main screen. Perform a drug look-up procedure to confirm that the new compound has been correctly added to the computer system.

a. Click on the **Drug** button on the left side of the screen.

b. Click the **Find** 🔍 icon located at the top left of the toolbar.

c. The *Drug Name Lookup* dialog box appears. Type in the label name of the new compound.

Enter *ANN,* or use the Quick Code you selected—*ANNAAW*
for Anna's Antiwrinkle Cream.

d. Select the correct compound from the list by clicking on the drug name. Click **OK**.

e. Read through the *Drugs* form to check for accuracy. Click the **Compound Drug Ingredients** tab at the bottom of the screen to verify the ingredients.

Print the screen, and save it for your instructor.

f. Click the **Close** 🔳 icon on the top right of the toolbar to clear the screen.

QUICK CHALLENGE

Fill in the medication order for the compound entered in the Lab. Use the following prescription for patient and prescriber information. You will then process the prescription for the individual patient and print a label.

 LAB TIP

Once the compound is entered in the database, fill a prescription using the quick code you selected for the compound. This will be the prescribed drug for the patient.

Dr. James Furman
3345 Atrium Drive
Albany, NY 12205
Office: (518) 555-4677
Fax: (518) 555-4679

Date: _____7/30/2017_____

Patient Name: ___Marjorie Davidson___

Address: ___27 Bradford Street, Newton, MA 02456___

℞

Anna's Antiwrinkle Cream
Tretinoin 0.05% cream, 2.5 g
SWFI 0.02 mL

Refill: ___0___

DEA: AF5190688

Dr. J. Furman
M.D.

LAB 23

Preparing and Processing Ointments

▪ Introduction

Extemporaneous compounding or *nonsterile compounding* includes preparing ointments. An ointment is an oil-in-water (O/W) preparation and is designed to stay on the surface of the skin as a barrier. It will have a smooth to a slightly greasy feel and will typically be compounded by adding powders, other ointments, or solutions to a base and then incorporating (mixing) them together with a spatula.

A ***master formula record (FR)*** is used as a recipe and includes all of the required ingredients and instructions for preparation and documentation. If the compound is written for a specific patient on a prescription, then the directions may vary by physician. In addition to the master FR, a ***compounding record (CR)*** or ***log*** will also be generated (on completion of the preparation) to provide a record of the compound itself. This CR will include information such as the prescription number, each ingredient's information, and who made the compound and who checked it.

A ***safety data sheet (SDS)*** is available for each active ingredient and should be included as part of the documentation for every compound made.

▪ Lab Objectives

In this Lab, you will:

- Demonstrate the skills required for interpreting, calculating, and preparing a compounded ointment from a prescription.
- Prepare an electronic label from a prescription for a medication.
- Complete a repackaging log.
- Identify special requirements for ointment medications, including the use of equipment, techniques, and patient directions for storage.
- Demonstrate ethics, adhere to patient privacy, and work as a team member in a simulated laboratory scenario.

ASHP goals: 7, 11, 12, 16, 18, 21, 22, 25, 26, 27, 29, 33, 35, 36, 41, and 44.

▪ Scenario

In your pharmacy today, you have been assigned to the compounding section. Once calculations are performed and a label is prepared, you must gather the equipment and prepare the ointment compound. The final product must be recorded, have proper labeling, and be checked at each key interval, as determined by the master FR or recipe.

▪ Pre Lab Information

Using the Visual SuperScript database, as well as the prescriptions, medications, and supplies provided, review the process for flavoring and reconstituting your prescription. Use a reference source to find storage information (beyond use date [BUD]), and identify any auxiliary labels or special instructions required before entering the prescription.

▪ Student Directions

Estimated completion time: 30 minutes

Interpret the following prescription, including all calculations and the day's supply.

Dr. Shane Dalton
1901 W. Hemlock Street
Hyde Park, MA 02136
Office: (617) 555-6000
Fax: (617) 555-6002

Date: _____7/15/2017_____

Patient Name: ___Marjorie Davidson___

Address: ___27 Bradford Street, Newton, MA___

℞

0.2% Nitr ointment 60 g
Apply ½-inch q 8 hrs
Refill: ___3___ *Use application papers and gloves

DEA: AD1234563

Dr. S. Dalton
M.D.

0.2% Nitroglycerin (Nitro) ointment compound

   2 oz = 60 g

   $0.2\% \times 60\ g = 2\% \times x\ g$

   Solve for x g and you get 6 g

   You will need 6 g of the 2% nitro ointment and 54 g of base.

Two tubes of simulated Nitroglycerin ointment 2% 3 g
Simulated Nitroglycerin application papers #50 pkg

 LAB TIP

Use your **master FR** to gather the needed ingredients and supplies to prepare this medication.

STEPS TO PREPARE AND PROCESS COMPOUNDED OINTMENTS

1. Using Lab 22 as a reference, enter the compounded ointment and prepare a prescription for Ms. Davidson.

2. After completing the information on the **DRUG AND PACKAGING** form, use the following directions to enter the required ingredients for the ointment.

3. Key in the first few letters of the desired drug ingredient. Select the correct drug from the list by clicking on the drug name. Click **OK**.

Search for *CMPNITR* for Nitroglycern (Nitro) 2% 3 g ointment.
Select the 3 g package size for this drug.

 LAB TIP

Remember to search using the first two letters of the desired drug, and always review the dose and package size for the item you choose. Once this is done, you will charge for the amount needed to make your compound. In this case, you will need to use 6 g or less (two in-stock 3-g tubes), and you will charge for a total of 6 g needed to make the medication.

4. In the *Compound Drug Ingredients* dialog box, type in the correct quantity of drug (in grams) that you will need.

For this ingredient, you will need 6 g (based on calculations performed).
This will be two tubes.

5. Click the **SAVE** 💾 icon on the bottom of the *Compound Drug Ingredients* dialog box.

Enter *DD* for Demo Dose SIMBASE ointment 500 g.

6. In the *Compound Drug Ingredients* dialog box, type in the correct quantity of drug (in grams) that you will need.

You will need to charge for 54 g (based on calculations performed).

 LAB TIP

If you have more ingredients, add each ingredient one at a time by clicking on the **NEW** 🗋 icon located at the bottom right of the *Drugs* form. Review the steps in this Lab to add each ingredient.

7. Once all of the ingredients are added, click the **CLOSE** 🔌 icon at the top right of the toolbar. The compound is now saved.

8. You are now returned to the main screen. Perform a drug look-up procedure to confirm that the new compound has been correctly added to the computer system.

   a. Click on the **DRUG** button on the left side of the screen.
   b. Click the **FIND** 🔍 icon located at the top left of the toolbar.
   c. The *Drug Name Lookup* dialog box appears. Type in the label name of the new compound.

   Enter *MDNITR 0.2% 60 g* for your compound.

   d. Select the correct compound from the list by clicking on the drug name. Click **OK**.
   e. Read through the *Drugs* form to check for accuracy.

   Print the screen, and save it for your instructor.

   f. Click the **CLOSE** 🔌 icon at the top right of the toolbar to clear the screen.

STEPS TO PREPARE THE LABEL FOR A COMPOUNDED PRESCRIPTION

1. Once the compound is entered in the database, fill a prescription using the directions in Lab 6 and the quick code you selected for the compound. This will be the prescribed drug for the patient.

   Enter Quick code *BDNITR 0.2% 60 g*.

2. Type in the appropriate days' supply in the **PRESCRIBED DAYS SUPPLY** data entry field.

   Enter *30* for the days' supply.

3. Once the product is compounded, you will need to apply a ***For topical use only*** sticker along with the patient label on the container.

1. Once the labels are printed, retrieve the ingredients needed from the shelf.
2. Follow the master FR provided, and complete each step as it is written.

Master Formula Record
(for training purposes only)

Nitroglycern (Nitr) 0.2% 60 g cream

INGREDIENT/DRUG	AMOUNT
Demo Dose Nitroglycern (Nitr Derm) 2% 3 g ointment	6 gm
DD SIMBASE ointment 500 g	54 gm

Equipment and supplies needed

Scale   Gloves
Spatula—minimum 8 in.   Ointment container 2 oz
Weighing boats (2) MED   Alcohol and wipes

NOTE: It is recommended that you follow USP <795> recommendations for potency testing that states "each preparation shall contain not less than 90.0% and not more than 110.0% of the theoretically calculated and labeled quantity of active ingredient." To provide some guidance in this area, use the "percentage of error" formula to calculate potency if required by your Instructor.

This is for simulation training purposes only and has not been tested in a PCCA lab, and all required steps in process should be verified by Instructor.

Suggested Compounding Procedures

1. Perform calculations and measure each ingredient separately with a 10% excess (Nitr in boat) and (SIMBASE in boat).
   NOTE: Some material may be lost due to sticking to sides of container. Making 10% more will provide enough to measure the full 60 gm needed.
2. Have your Instructor check weights of each.
3. Using the spatula, place the SIMBASE ointment and Nitr on the ointment slab.
4. Using spatulation, combine the two ingredients completely.
5. Once mixed, pack the ointment jar using the spatula.
   NOTE: Gather ointment on the spatula tip and slide it into the bottom of the jar, continuing this process until all material is inside and sides near top are clean. Using the flat side of spatula, smooth top of material in jar and clean all material from the spatula and the ointment slab.
6. Assign a BUD after compounding following USP 795 guidelines, and complete compounding record/log. Estimated to be 30 days or less.

Warning: Safety precautions should be taken when compounding and using equipment. Follow all laboratory and product safety guidelines, and wear appropriate personal protective equipment.

 LAB TIP

Each ingredient has a specific lot number, bar code, and expiration date provided by the U.S. Food and Drug Administration (FDA). To verify that the correct medication is being compounded, this number must match the master FR list of ingredients and the compounding record once finished.

3. Prepare the **CR** with all required information. An editable version of the CR is available on the Evolve Resources site.

Compounding Record Drug _____ Date _____

Prescription Number or ID Assigned	Master FR Record # Used	Name and Strength of Compound	Quantity	Actual Net Measurements	Expiration Date	MFG Lot Number	MFG Expiration Date	BUD Assigned	Date Packaged	Tech Initials	RPh Initials

Attach a prescription/patient label if applicable.

ID, Identification; *FR,* formula record; *MFG,* manufacturer; *BUD,* beyond use date; *RPh,* registered pharmacist.

4. Locate the **SDS** for all ingredients using http://chemicalsafety.com/sds/.

5. Once the pharmacist has completed the verification process, simulate the dispensing to include customer interaction, processing the sale, and final packaging.

RESOURCES

Allen LV, Adejare A, Desselle SP, Felton LA (eds): *Remington: the science and practice of pharmacy*, ed 22, London, 2013, Pharmaceutical Press.

Mosby's drug reference for health professions, ed 4, St Louis, 2014, Mosby.

LAB 24

Preparing and Processing Creams

▪ Introduction

Extemporaneous compounding or *nonsterile compounding* includes preparing creams. A *water-in-oil* (W/O) preparation is designed to soak into or penetrate the skin. It will have a smooth, slightly cool feel and will typically be compounded by adding other creams, powders, or solutions to a base and incorporating (mixing) them together with a spatula.

A ***master formula record (FR)*** is used as a recipe and includes all the required ingredients and instructions for preparation and documentation. If the compound is written for a specific patient on a prescription, then the directions may vary by physician. In addition to the master FR, a ***compounding record (CR) or log*** will also be generated (on completion of the preparation) to provide a record of the compound itself. This CR will include information such as the prescription number, each ingredient's information, and who made the compound and who checked it.

A ***safety data sheet (SDS)*** is available for each active ingredient and should be included as part of the documentation for every compound made.

▪ Lab Objectives

In this Lab, you will:

- Demonstrate the skills required for interpreting, calculating, and preparing a cream compound from a prescription.
- Prepare an electronic label from a prescription for a cream medication.
- Complete a repackaging log.
- Identify special requirements for cream medications, including the use of equipment, techniques, and patient directions for storage.
- Demonstrate ethics, adhere to patient privacy, and work as a team member in a simulated laboratory scenario.

ASHP goals: 7, 11, 12, 16, 18, 21, 22, 25, 26, 27, 29, 33, 35, 36, 41, and 44.

▪ Scenario

In your pharmacy today, you have been assigned to the compounding section. Once calculations are performed and a label is prepared, you must gather the equipment and prepare the cream. The final product must be recorded, have proper labeling, and be checked at each key interval, as determined by the master FR or recipe.

▪ Pre Lab Information

Using the Visual SuperScript database, as well as the prescriptions, medications, and supplies provided, review the process for flavoring and reconstituting your prescription. Use a reference source to find storage information (beyond use date [BUD]), and identify any auxiliary labels or special instructions required before entering the prescription.

Estimated completion time: 30 minutes

Dr. Isabel Fairchild
1901 W. Hemlock Street
Hyde Park, MA 02136
Office: (617) 555-4600
Fax: (617) 555-4602

Date: ___3/23/2017___

Patient Name: ___Wilma Flintstone___

Address: ___123 Bedrock Hwy, Waltham, MA 02454___

Rx

3.3% Simulated Progesteron cream 60 g
Apply bid

Refill: ___0___

DEA: MF1234688

Dr. I. Fairchild
M.D.

Interpret the above prescription, including all calculations and the days' supply.

Compound 3.3% Simulated Progesteron cream 60 g

3.3% is 33.3 mg per milliliter or gram

$$\frac{33.3 \text{ mg}}{\text{mL}} = \frac{x}{60 \text{ mL}} = 1.99 \text{ g}$$

1.99 g of the powder is needed, therefore the remainder is the base. Take the difference to get the amount: 60 g – 1.98 = 58 g of cream base.

You will need DD Progesteron and DD SIMBASE CREAM.

DD POWDER Progesteron (Prometrim) 100 g
DD SIMBASE CREAM 500 g

 LAB TIP

Use your **master FR** to gather the needed ingredients and supplies to prepare this medication.

STEPS TO PREPARE AND PROCESS CREAMS

1. Using Lab 22 as a reference, enter the compounded cream and prepare a prescription for Ms. Flintstone.

2. After completing the information on the **DRUG AND PACKAGING** form, use the following directions to enter the required ingredients for the cream.

3. Key in the first few letters of the desired drug ingredient. Select the correct drug from the list by clicking on the drug name. Click **OK**.

Search for *DD* for SIMBASE POWDER Progesteron (Prometrim) 100 g.
Select the correct package size (100 g for this drug).

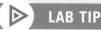 **LAB TIP**

Remember to search using the first two letters of the desired drug, and always review the dose and package size for the item you choose. Once this is done, you will charge for the amount needed to make your compound.

4. In the *Compound Drug Ingredients* dialog box, type in the correct quantity of drug (in grams) that you will need.

> **For this ingredient, you will need 1.99 g (based on calculations performed).**

5. Click the **SAVE** icon on the bottom of the *Compound Drug Ingredients* dialog box.

> **Enter *DD* for Demo Dose SIMBASE CREAM 500 g.**

6. In the *Compound Drug Ingredients* dialog box, type in the correct quantity of drug (in grams) that you will need.

> **You will need to charge for 58 g (based on calculations performed).**

▷ **LAB TIP**

If you have more ingredients, add each ingredient one at a time by clicking on the **NEW** ☐ icon located at the bottom right of the *Drugs* form. Review the steps in this Lab to add each ingredient.

7. Once all of the ingredients are added, click the **CLOSE** ▯◆ icon at the top right of the toolbar. The compound is now saved.

8. You are now returned to the main screen. Perform a drug look-up procedure to confirm that the new compound has been correctly added to the computer system.

　a. Click on the **DRUG** button on the left side of the screen.

　b. Click the **FIND** 🔍 icon located at the top left of the toolbar.

　c. The *Drug Name Lookup* dialog box appears. Type in the label name of the new compound.

> **Enter *PAProg3.3%60C* for your compound.**

　d. Select the correct compound from the list by clicking on the drug name. Click **OK**.

　e. Read through the *Drugs* form to check for accuracy.

> **Print the screen, and save it for your instructor.**

　f. Click the **CLOSE** ▯◆ icon on the top right of the toolbar to clear the screen.

STEPS TO PREPARE THE LABEL FOR A COMPOUNDED PRESCRIPTION

1. Once the compound is entered in the database, fill a prescription using the directions in Lab 6 and the quick code you selected for the compound. This will be the prescribed drug for the patient.

> **Enter Quick code *PAProg3.3%60C*.**

2. Type in the appropriate days' supply in the **PRESCRIBED DAYS SUPPLY** data entry field.

> **Enter *30* in the PRESCRIBED DAYS SUPPLY data entry field.**

3. Once the product is compounded, you will need to apply a ***For topical use only*** sticker along with the patient label on the container.

1. Once the labels are printed, retrieve the ingredients needed from the shelf.

 LAB TIP

Each ingredient has a specific lot number, bar code, and expiration date provided by the U.S. Food and Drug Administration (FDA). To verify that the correct medication is being compounded, this number must match the master FR list of ingredients and the compounding record once finished.

2. Follow the master FR provided, and complete each step as it is written.

Community Pharmacy Practice

Master Formula Record
(for training purposes only)
Progesteron 3.3% cream 60 g

INGREDIENT/DRUG	AMOUNT
DD POWDER Progesteron (Prometrim) 100 g	1.99 g
DD SIMBASE CREAM 500 g	58 g

Equipment and supplies needed

Scale
Spatulas—(2) 6-8 in.
Syringe adapter
Weighing boat LG
Alcohol and wipes

Gloves
60 mL syringes (2)
Syringe tip cap
Weighing papers (2 each)

NOTE: It is recommended that you follow USP <795> recommendations for potency testing, which states "each preparation shall contain not less than 90.0% and not more than 110.0% of the theoretically calculated and labeled quantity of active ingredient." To provide some guidance in this area, use the "percentage of error" formula to calculate potency, if required by the *Instructor*.

This Master Formula Record is for simulation training purposes only and has not been tested in a PCCA laboratory, and all required steps in the process should be verified by Instructor.

Suggested Compounding Procedures

1. Perform calculations, and measure each ingredient separately with a 10% excess (Progesteron on paper) and (SIMBASE in boat).
   NOTE: Some material may be lost attributable to sticking to sides or container. Making 10% more will provide enough to measure the full 60 g needed.
2. Have your *Instructor* check the weights of each.
3. Using the spatula, place the SIMBASE CREAM and Progesteron on a glass slab.
4. Using spatulation, gradually add powder to the base, and mix thoroughly. Combine the two ingredients completely.
5. Once mixed, pack the ointment jar using the spatula.
   NOTE: Gather cream on the spatula tip, and slide it into the bottom of the jar, continuing this process until all material is inside and sides near top are clean. Using the flat side of spatula, smooth top of material in jar and clean all material from the spatula and the ointment slab.
6. Assign a BUD after compounding following USP 795 guidelines, and complete the compounding record/log. Estimated to be 30 days or less.

Warning: *Safety precautions should be taken when compounding and using equipment. Follow all laboratory and product safety guidelines, and wear appropriate personal protective equipment.*

3. Prepare the **CR** with all required information.

Compounding Record   Drug _____   Date _____

Prescription Number or ID Assigned	Master FR Record # Used	Name and Strength of Compound	Quantity	Actual Net Measurements	Expiration Date	MFG Lot Number	MFG Expiration Date	BUD Assigned	Date Packaged	Tech Initials	RPh Initials

Attach a prescription/patient label if applicable.

ID, Identification; *FR,* formula record; *MFG,* manufacturer; *BUD,* beyond use date; *RPh,* registered pharmacist.

4. Locate the **SDS** for all ingredients by using www.pocketnurse.com.

5. Once the pharmacist has completed the verification process, simulate the dispensing to include customer interaction, processing the sale, and final packaging.

RESOURCES

Allen LV, Adejare A, Desselle SP, Felton LA (eds): *Remington: the science and practice of pharmacy*, ed 22, London, 2013, Pharmaceutical Press.

Mosby's drug reference for health professions, ed 4, St Louis, 2014, Mosby.

Pharmaceutical Compounding—Nonsterile Preparations. The United States Pharmacopeial Convention, 2014. Retrieved from http://www.usp.org/sites/default/files/usp_pdf/EN/gc795.pdf

The Pharmaceutics and Compounding Laboratory, University of North Carolina at Chapel Hill, Eshelman School of Pharmacy, 2015. Retrieved from http://pharmlabs.unc.edu/

LAB 25

Preparing and Processing Medicated Troches (Lozenges)

▪ Introduction

Extemporaneous compounding or *nonsterile compounding* includes preparing medicated troches (lozenges). A patient may be experiencing a mouth- or throat-related procedure, injury, or oral lesions from an infection such as yeast. The troche (lozenge) base is clear and can be mixed with lidocaine and can be sweetened, or flavored, and colored with medicated powders.

To compound this dosage form, the base is melted using a hot plate. The medication and any flavoring needed is then added and allowed to cool. After cooling, the mixture is poured into a mold and allowed to cool.

A *master formula record (FR)* is used as a recipe and includes all the required ingredients and instructions for preparation and documentation. If the compound is written for a specific patient on a prescription, then the directions may vary by physician. In addition to the master FR, a *compounding record (CR)* or *log* will also be generated (on completion of the preparation) to provide a record of the compound itself. This CR will include information such as the prescription number, each ingredient's information, and who made the compound and who checked it.

A *safety data sheet (SDS)* is available for each active ingredient and should be included as part of the documentation for every compound made.

▪ Lab Objectives

In this Lab, you will:

- Demonstrate the skills required for interpreting, calculating, and preparing a troche (lozenge) compound from a prescription.
- Prepare an electronic label from a prescription for a troche (lozenge) dosage form.
- Complete a repackaging log.
- Identify special requirements for troche (lozenge) medications, including the use of equipment, techniques, and patient directions for storage.
- Demonstrate ethics, adhere to patient privacy, and work as a team member in a simulated laboratory scenario.

ASHP goals: 7, 11, 12, 16, 18, 21, 22, 25, 26, 27, 29, 33, 35, 36, 41, and 44.

▪ Scenario

In your pharmacy today, you have been assigned to the compounding section. Once calculations are performed and a label is prepared, you must gather the equipment and prepare the troches. The final product must be recorded, have proper labeling, and be checked at each key interval, as determined by the master FR or recipe.

▪ Pre Lab Information

Using the Visual Superscript database, as well as the prescriptions, medications, and supplies provided, review the compounding process of your prescription. In this case, the physician has supplied the pharmacy with a standing recipe (master FR), and the prescription reflects only the medication and amount needed. The patient has severe mouth ulcers. Use a reference source to find storage information (beyond use date [BUD]), and identify any auxiliary labels or special instructions required before entering the prescription.

Estimated completion time: 30 minutes

Dr. Louise Clayton
645 S. Cedar Street
Cambridge, MA 02139
Office: (617) 555-4300
Fax: (617) 555-4302

Date: _____2/28/2017_____

Patient Name: ___Jason Moran___

Address: ___5534 W. Ash Street, Gloucester, MA 01930___

R **X**   API troches (lozenges) #10
        Hold the lozenge in the mouth and
Refill: __2__   allow to dissolve slowly and completely.

DEA: BC1234727

Dr. L. Clayton
M.D.

Interpret the above prescription, including all calculations and the days' supply.

API troche (lozenge) #10

 LAB TIP

Use your **master FR** at the end of this Lab to gather the needed ingredients and supplies to prepare this medication. The ingredient amounts have been already provided for making 10 troches; therefore you will calculate the amount needed for each ingredient. API means **active pharmaceutical ingredient** and simulates the medication lozenge in this activity.

DD SIMBASE Powder 500 g
DD POWDER Steviosid (Stevi) 500 g
DD SIMBASE LOLLIPOP 500 g, and flavor of your choice:
  DD Orange flavor 120 mL
  DD Grape flavor 120 mL
  DD Bubblegum flavor 120 mL

STEPS TO PREPARE AND PROCESS TROCHES

1. Using Lab 22 as a reference, enter the compounded troche and prepare a prescription for Jason.

2. After completing the information on the **DRUG AND PACKAGING** form, use the following directions to enter the required ingredients for the troche.

3. Key in the first few letters of the desired drug ingredient. Select the correct drug from the list by clicking on the drug name. Click **OK**.

Search for *DD* for SIMBASE Powder 500 g.
Select the 500 g for this drug.

LAB TIP

Remember to search using the first two letters of the desired drug, and always review the dose and package size for the item you choose. Once this is done, you will charge for the amount needed to make your compound. In this case, you will need to use 0.2 g or less per the master FR, and you will charge for a total of 0.2 g needed to make the medication.

4. In the *Compound Drug Ingredients* dialog box, type in the correct quantity of drug (in grams) that you will need.

For this ingredient, you will need 0.2 g per the master FR.

 LAB TIP

Continue to enter the other ingredients, one at a time, by clicking on the **NEW** [icon] icon located at the bottom right of the *Drugs* form. Review the steps in this Lab to add each ingredient.

5. Once all of the ingredients are added, click the **CLOSE** [icon] icon at the top right of the toolbar. The compound is now saved.

6. You are now returned to the main screen. Perform a drug look-up procedure to confirm that the new compound has been correctly added to the computer system.

   a. Click on the **DRUG** button on the left side of the screen.

   b. Click the **FIND** [icon] icon located at the top left of the toolbar.

   c. The *Drug Name Lookup* dialog box appears. Type in the label name of the new compound.

   Enter *API TROCHE* for your compound.

   d. Select the correct compound from the list by clicking on the drug name. Click **OK**.

   e. Read through the *Drugs* form to check for accuracy.

   Print the screen, and save it for your instructor.

   f. Click the **CLOSE** [icon] icon on the top right of the toolbar to clear the screen.

STEPS TO PREPARE THE LABEL FOR A COMPOUNDED PRESCRIPTION

1. Once the compound is entered in the database, fill a prescription using the directions in Lab 6 and the quick code you selected for the compound. This will be the prescribed drug for the patient.

Enter Quick code *API TROCHE*.

2. Type in the appropriate days' supply in the **PRESCRIBED DAYS SUPPLY** data entry field.

Enter *2* in the PRESCRIBED DAYS SUPPLY data entry field.

3. Once the product is compounded, you will need to apply a ***Do Not Refrigerate*** sticker along with the patient label on the container.

STEPS FOR THE PREPARATION OF A TROCHE (LOZENGE) PROCESS

1. Once the labels are printed, retrieve the ingredients needed from the shelf.

LAB TIP

Each ingredient has a specific lot number, bar code, and expiration date provided by the U.S. Food and Drug Administration (FDA). To verify that the correct medication is being compounded, this number must match the master FR list of ingredients and the compounding record once finished.

2. Follow the master FR provided, and complete each step as it is written.

Compounding Record   Drug _____   Date _____

Prescription Number or ID Assigned	Master FR Record # Used	Name and Strength of Compound	Quantity	Actual Net Measurements	Expiration Date	MFG Lot Number	MFG Expiration Date	BUD Assigned	Date Packaged	Tech Initials	RPh Initials

Attach a prescription/patient label if applicable.
ID, Identification; *FR,* formula record; *MFG,* manufacturer; *BUD,* beyond use date; *RPh,* registered pharmacist.

3. Prepare the CR with all required information.

4. Locate the **SDS** for all ingredients by using www.pocketnurse.com.

5. Once the pharmacist has completed the verification process, simulate the dispensing to include customer interaction, processing the sale, and final packaging.

RESOURCES

Allen LV, Adejare A, Desselle SP, Felton LA (eds): *Remington: the science and practice of pharmacy*, ed 22, London, 2013, Pharmaceutical Press.

Mosby's drug reference for health professions, ed 4, St Louis, 2014, Mosby.

Pharmaceutical Compounding—Nonsterile Preparations. The United States Pharmacopeial Convention, 2014. Retrieved from http://www.usp.org/sites/default/files/usp_pdf/EN/gc795.pdf

The Pharmaceutics and Compounding Laboratory, University of North Carolina at Chapel Hill Eshelman School of Pharmacy, 2015. Retrieved from http://pharmlabs.unc.edu/

LAB 26

Preparing and Processing Compounded Oral Liquids

■ Introduction

Extemporaneous compounding or *nonsterile compounding* includes preparing liquids, such as solutions or suspensions. A physician may order a specific medication that is made up of several liquid medications and give it a known name, or the pharmacy may have a standard recipe to follow for preparing a compounded liquid. A **master formula record (FR)** is used as a recipe and includes all the required ingredients and instructions for preparation and documentation. If the compound is written for a specific patient on a prescription, then the directions may vary by physician. In addition to the master FR, a **compounding record (CR)** or **log** will also be generated (on completion of the preparation) to provide a record of the compound itself. This CR will include information such as the prescription number, each ingredient's information, and who made the compound and who checked it.

A **safety data sheet (SDS)** is available for each active ingredient and should be included as part of the documentation for every compound made.

■ Lab Objectives

In this Lab, you will:

- Demonstrate the skills required for interpreting, calculating, and preparing an compounded oral liquid from a prescription.
- Prepare an electronic label from a prescription for a compounded oral medication.
- Complete a repackaging log.
- Identify special requirements for compounded oral liquid medications, including the use of equipment, techniques, and patient directions for storage.
- Demonstrate ethics, adhere to patient privacy, and work as a team member in a simulated laboratory scenario.

ASHP goals: 7, 11, 12, 16, 18, 21, 22, 25, 26, 27, 29, 33, 35, 36, 41, and 44.

■ Scenario

In your pharmacy today, you have been assigned to the compounding section. Once calculations are performed and a label is prepared, you must gather the equipment and prepare the oral liquid compound. The final product must be recorded, have proper labeling, and be checked at each key interval, as determined by the master FR or recipe.

■ Pre Lab Information

Using the Visual SuperScript database, as well as the prescriptions, medications, and supplies provided, review the process for flavoring and measuring liquids for (reading a meniscus) for your prescription. Use a reference source to find storage information (beyond use date [BUD]), and identify any auxiliary labels or special instructions required before entering the prescription.

Estimated completion time: 30 minutes

Interpret the following prescription, including all calculations and the days' supply. **The master FR has provided amounts of each ingredient for this compound.**

Dr. Isabel Fairchild   **Date:** _____10/14/2017_____
1901 W. Hemlock Street
Hyde Park, MA 02136
Office: (617) 555-4600
Fax: (617) 555-4602

Patient Name: ___Herbert Beard___

Address: ___452 Oakwood Drive, Waltham, MA 02454___

℞ Magic Mouthwash (simulated) 240 mL
Swish and swallow bid

Refill: ___0___ Label 06-93-1337N

DEA: MF1234688

Dr. I. Fairchild
M.D.

 LAB TIP

Use your **master FR** to gather the needed ingredients and supplies to prepare this medication. Check the expiration dates.

DD DiphenhydrAMIN (Benadrl) 12.5 mg/5 mL 473 mL

DD Alm/Mg/Simethicon 200 mg/mL (Maalx) 473 mL

DD Triamcinolon acet (Nystatn) 100,000 units/mL suspension 473 mL

DD HCI 2% oral topical Viscous solution 100 mL

STEPS TO PREPARE AND PROCESS COMPOUNDED ORAL LIQUIDS

1. Using Lab 22 as a reference, enter the compounded oral liquid and prepare a prescription for Mr. Beard.

2. After completing the information on the **DRUG AND PACKAGING** form, use the following directions to enter the required ingredients for the oral liquid.

3. Key in the first few letters of the desired drug ingredient. Select the correct drug from the list by clicking on the drug name. Click **OK**.

> **Search *DD* for DiphenhydrAMIN (Benadrl) 12.5 mg/5 mL 473 mL.**
> **Select the 480 mL for package size for this drug.**

LAB TIP

Remember to search using first two letters of the desired drug, and always review the dose and package size for the item you choose. Once this is done, you will charge for the amount needed for the compound you are making. In this case, you will need to use 60 mL out of the in-stock 480-mL bottle, and you will only charge for the 60 mL needed to make the medication

4. In the *Compound Drug Ingredients* dialog box, type in the correct quantity of drug (in milliliters) that you will need.

   For this ingredient, you will need 60 mL (based on calculations performed).

5. Click the **Save** 💾 icon on the bottom of the *Compound Drug Ingredients* dialog box.

LAB TIP

Continue to add the other ingredients one at a time by clicking on the **New** 🗋 icon located at the bottom right of the *Drugs* form. Review the steps in this Lab to add each ingredient.

6. Once all of the ingredients are added, click the **Close** 🚪 icon at the top right of the toolbar. The compound is now saved.

7. You are now returned to the main screen. Perform a drug look-up procedure to confirm that the new compound has been correctly added to the computer system.

   a. Click on the **Drug** button on the left side of the screen.

   b. Click the **Find** 🔍 icon located at the top left of the toolbar.

   c. The *Drug Name Lookup* dialog box appears. Type in the label name of the new compound.

      Enter *KAMAGCMW240* for your compound.

   d. Select the correct compound from the list by clicking on the drug name. Click **OK**.

   e. Read through the *Drugs* form to check for accuracy.

      Print the screen, and save it for your instructor.

   f. Click the **Close** 🚪 icon on the top right of the toolbar to clear the screen.

STUDENT DIRECTIONS FOR PREPARING A LABEL FOR A COMPOUND PRESCRIPTION

1. Once the compound is entered in the database, fill a prescription using the directions in Lab 6 and the quick code you selected for the compound. This will be the prescribed drug for the patient.

   Enter Quick code *KAMAGCMW240*.

LAB TIP

The **Quick Code** is the code you gave the drug when it was entered as a compound.

2. Type in the appropriate days' supply in the **Prescribed Days Supply** data entry field.

   Enter *14* for the days' supply.

3. Once the product is compounded, you will need to apply a ***Shake well*** sticker along with the patient label on the container.

STEPS FOR THE PREPARATION OF A COMPOUNDED ORAL SUSPENSION PROCESS

1. Once the labels are printed, retrieve the ingredients needed from the shelf.

 LAB TIP

Each ingredient has a specific lot number, bar code, and expiration date provided by the U.S. Food and Drug Administration (FDA). To verify that the correct medication is being compounded, this number must match the master FR list of ingredients and the compounding record once finished.

2. Follow the master FR provided, and complete each step as it is written.

Master Formula Record
(for training purposes only)

Magc Mouthwash 240 mL

INGREDIENT/DRUG	AMOUNT
DD Lidocain HCl 2% oral topical Viscous solution 100 mL	60 mL
DD DiphenhydrAMIN (Benadrl) 12.5 mg/5 mL 473 mL	60 mL
DD Alm/Mg/Simethicon 200 mg/mL (Maalx) 473 mL	60 mL
DD Triamcinolon acet (Nystatn) 100,000 units/mL suspension 473 mL	60 mL

Equipment and Supplies needed

Graduated cylinders (4) 100 mL
8 oz amber bottle

NOTE: It is recommended that you follow USP <795> recommendations for potency testing, which states "each preparation shall contain not less than 90.0% and not more than 110.0% of the theoretically calculated and labeled quantity of active ingredient." To provide some guidance in this area, use the "percentage of error" formula to calculate potency, if required by your *Instructor*.

This Master Formula Record is for simulation training purposes only and has not been tested in a PCCA laboratory, and all required steps in the process should be verified by Instructor.

Suggested Compounding Procedures

1. Measure each ingredient (reading the meniscus) separately with individual graduated cylinders.
   NOTE: For thicker liquids, try to ring the center of the container when measuring so it does not stick to the outer surfaces. This will make it easier to measure the amount needed once they sit a few minutes.
2. Have your student partner and Instructor check amounts of each
3. Using the 8 oz container, add each liquid individually and mix.
4. Assign a BUD after compounding following USP 795 guidelines and complete compounding record/log. Estimated to be 14 days or less.

Warning: Safety precautions should be taken when compounding and using equipment. Follow all laboratory and product safety guidelines and wear appropriate personal protective equipment.

3. Prepare the **CR** with all required information.

Compounding Record　　　　Drug _____　　　　Date _____

Prescription Number or ID Assigned	Master FR Record # Used	Name and Strength of Compound	Quantity	Actual Net Measurements	Expiration Date	MFG Lot Number	MFG Expiration Date	BUD Assigned	Date Packaged	Tech Initials	RPh Initials

Attach a prescription/patient label if applicable.
ID, Identification; *FR,* formula record; *MFG,* manufacturer; *BUD,* beyond use date; *RPh,* registered pharmacist.

4. Locate the **SDS** for all ingredients using www.pocketnurse.com.

5. Once the pharmacist has completed the verification process, simulate the dispensing to include customer interaction, processing the sale, and final packaging.

RESOURCES

Allen LV, Adejare A, Desselle SP, Felton LA (eds): *Remington: the science and practice of pharmacy,* ed 22, London, 2013, Pharmaceutical Press.

Mosby's drug reference for health professions, ed 4, St Louis, 2014, Mosby.

Pharmaceutical Compounding—Nonsterile Preparations. The United States Pharmacopeial Convention, 2014. Retrieved from http://www.usp.org/sites/default/files/usp_pdf/EN/gc795.pdf

The Pharmaceutics and Compounding Laboratory, University of North Carolina at Chapel Hill, Eshelman School of Pharmacy, 2015. Retrieved from http://pharmlabs.unc.edu/

LAB 27

Preparing and Processing Medicated Lollipops

▪ Introduction

Extemporaneous compounding or *nonsterile compounding* includes preparing medicated lollipops. A patient may be experiencing a mouth- or throat-related procedure, injury, or oral lesion that requires numbing or a pain medication. The lollipop base is clear and can be mixed with medicated powders such as lidocaine or a pain medication and can be sweetened, flavored, and colored.

To compound this dosage form, the base is melted using a hot plate. The medication and any flavoring needed is then added and allowed to cool. After cooling, the mixture is poured into a mold and allowed to cool.

A *master formula record (FR)* is used as a recipe and includes all the required ingredients and instructions for preparation and documentation. If the compound is written for a specific patient on a prescription, then the directions may vary by physician. In addition to the master FR, a *compounding record (CR)* or *log* will also be generated (on completion of the preparation) to provide a record of the compound itself. This CR will include information such as the prescription number, each ingredient's information, and who made the compound and who checked it.

A *safety data sheet (SDS)* is available for each active ingredient and should be included as part of the documentation for every compound made.

▪ Lab Objectives

In this Lab, you will:

- Demonstrate the skills required for interpreting, calculating, and preparing a lollipop compound from a prescription.
- Prepare an electronic label from a prescription for a lollipop dosage form.
- Complete a repackaging log.
- Identify special requirements for lollipop medications, including the use of equipment, techniques, and patient directions for storage.
- Demonstrate ethics, adhere to patient privacy, and work as a team member in a simulated laboratory scenario.

ASHP goals: 7, 11, 12, 16, 18, 21, 22, 25, 26, 27, 29, 33, 35, 36, 41, and 44.

▪ Scenario

In your pharmacy today, you have been assigned to the compounding section. Once calculations are performed and a label is prepared, you must gather the equipment and prepare the lollipop compound. The final product must be recorded, have proper labeling, and be checked at each key interval, as determined by the master FR or recipe.

▪ Pre Lab Information

Using the Visual Superscript database, as well as the prescriptions, medications, and supplies provided, review the compounding process of your prescription. In this case, the physician has supplied the pharmacy with a standing recipe (master FR), and the prescription reflects only the medication and amount needed. The patient has postoperative tonsillitis. Use a reference source to find storage information (beyond use date [BUD]), and identify any auxiliary labels or special instructions required before entering the prescription.

Estimated completion time: 30 minutes

Interpret the following prescription, including all calculations and the days' supply.

Dr. Louise Clayton
645 S. Cedar Street
Cambridge, MA 02139
Office: (617) 555-4300
Fax: (617) 555-4302

Date: _____10/14/2017_____

Patient Name: __Jason Moran__

Address: ___5534 W. Ash Street, Gloucester, MA 01930___

R̶x

Acetaminophn lollipops #10
Suck on lollipop for 10-15 seconds,
then stop. May repeat every 2-3 hours.

Refill: __0__

DEA: BC1234727

Dr. L. Clayton
M.D.

Acetaminophen lollipops #10
If the patient can use one every 2 to 3 hours, then this amount would last only a little less than 1 day.

 LAB TIP

Use your **master FR** to gather the needed ingredients and supplies to prepare this medication. The ingredient amounts have been already provided for making 10 lollipops; therefore you will calculate the amount needed for each ingredient.

DD Acetaminophn–APAP powder 100 g
DD POWDER Steviosid 100 g
DD Grape flavor 120 mL
DD SIMBASE LOLLIPOP 500 g

STEPS TO PREPARE AND PROCESS MEDICATED LOLLIPOPS

1. Using Lab 22 as a reference, enter the medicated lollipop and prepare a prescription for Jason.

2. After completing the information on the **DRUG AND PACKAGING** form, use the following directions to enter the required ingredients for the medicated lollipop.

3. Key in the first few letters of the desired drug ingredient. Select the correct drug from the list by clicking on the drug name. Click **OK**.

Search for *DD* for DD Acetaminophn–APAP powder 100 g.
Select the 500 g for this drug.

LAB TIP

Remember to search using the first two letters of the desired drug, and always review the dose and package size for the item you choose. Once this is done, you will charge for the amount needed to make your compound. In this case, you will need to use 0.2 g and less per the master FR, and you will charge a total of 0.2 g needed to make the medication.

4. In the *Compound Drug Ingredients* dialog box, type in the correct quantity of drug (in grams) that you will need.

For this ingredient, you will need 0.2 g per the master FR.

 LAB TIP

Continue to enter the other ingredients, one at a time, by clicking on the **NEW** 📄 icon located at the bottom right of the *Drugs* form. Review the steps in this Lab to add each ingredient.

5. Once all of the ingredients are added, click the **CLOSE** 🔲 icon on the top right of the toolbar. The compound is now saved.

6. You are now returned to the main screen. Perform a drug look-up procedure to confirm that the new compound has been correctly added to the computer system.

    a. Click on the Drug button on the left side of the screen.

    b. Click the **FIND** 🔍 icon located at the top left of the toolbar.

    c. The *Drug Name Lookup* dialog box appears. Type in the label name of the new compound.

        Enter *APAP LOL* for your compound.

    d. Select the correct compound from the list by clicking on the drug name. Click **OK**.

    e. Read through the *Drugs* form to check for accuracy.

        Print the screen, and save it for your instructor.

    f. Click the **CLOSE** 🔲 icon on the top right of the toolbar to clear the screen.

STEPS TO PREPARE THE LABEL FOR A COMPOUNDED PRESCRIPTION

1. Once the compound is entered in the database, fill a prescription using the directions in Lab 6 and the quick code you selected for the compound. This will be the prescribed drug for the patient.

    Enter Quick code *APAP LOL*.

2. Type in the appropriate days' supply in the **PRESCRIBED DAYS SUPPLY** data entry field.

    Enter *1* in the PRESCRIBED DAYS SUPPLY data entry field.

3. Once the product is compounded, you will need to apply a ***Do Not Refrigerate*** sticker along with the patient label on the container.

1. Once the labels are printed, retrieve the ingredients needed from the shelf.

2. Follow the master FR provided, and complete each step as it is written.

Master Formula Record
(for training purposes only)

Demo Dose API Lollipops

INGREDIENT/DRUG	AMOUNT
DD Acetaminophn-APAP powder	100 g
DD Steviosid	0.12 g
DD SIMBASE lollipop	0.15 g
DD grape flavor	0.3 mL
DD color (violet)	1-2 gtts

Equipment and supplies needed

Scale
Oven mitt
Gloves
Measuring device (syringe) 1 mL
Lozenge mold
Alcohol and wipes

Stirring hotplate and rod
Boats/weighing papers
Spatula—minimum 8 in.
Dropper
Cooking (spray) oil

NOTE: It is recommended that you follow USP <795> recommendations for potency testing, which states "each preparation shall contain not less than 90.0% and not more than 110.0% of the theoretically calculated and labeled quantity of active ingredient." To provide some guidance in this area, use the "percentage of error" formula to calculate potency, if required by the *Instructor*.

This Master Formula Record is for simulation training purposes only and has not been tested in a PCCA laboratory, and all required steps in the process should be verified by the Instructor.

Suggested Compounding Procedures

1. Melt the SIMBASE lollipop base in a hot water bath, stirring frequently.
2. Triturate the powders in a mortar using geometric dilution.
3. Slowly add the powders into the melted base, and stir by hand until evenly dispersed.
4. As soon as evenly mixed, flavoring and/or coloring should be added, stir, and remove from heat.
   NOTE: Make sure you have the mold ready (sprayed with cooking oil) before removing from heat.
5. Pour into a mold, and spread mixture with spatula, if needed.
6. Allow to cool at room temperature.
7. Once room temperature, place in refrigerator.
8. Package and label (using gloves).
9. Assign a BUD after compounding, following USP 795 guidelines, and complete the compounding record/log. Estimated to be 14 days or less.

Warning: *Safety precautions should be taken when compounding and using equipment. Follow all laboratory and product safety guidelines, and wear appropriate personal protective equipment.*

LAB TIP

Each ingredient has a specific lot number, bar code, and expiration date provided by the U.S. Food and Drug Administration (FDA). To verify that the correct medication is being compounded, this number must match the master FR list of ingredients and the compounding record once finished.

3. Prepare the CR with all required information.

Compounding Record   Drug _____   Date _____

Prescription Number or ID Assigned	Master FR Record # Used	Name and Strength of Compound	Quantity	Actual Net Measurements	Expiration Date	MFG Lot Number	MFG Expiration Date	BUD Assigned	Date Packaged	Tech Initials	RPh Initials

Attach a prescription/patient label if applicable.
ID, Identification; *FR*, formula record; *MFG*, manufacturer; *BUD*, beyond use date; *RPh*, registered pharmacist.

4. Locate the **SDS** for all ingredients using www.pocketnurse.com.

5. Once the pharmacist has completed the verification process, simulate the dispensing to include customer interaction, processing the sale, and final packaging.

RESOURCES

Allen LV, Adejare A, Desselle SP, Felton LA (eds): *Remington: the science and practice of pharmacy*, ed 22, London, 2013, Pharmaceutical Press.

Mosby's drug reference for health professions, ed 4, St Louis, 2014, Mosby.

Pharmaceutical Compounding—Nonsterile Preparations. The United States Pharmacopeial Convention, 2014. Retrieved from http://www.usp.org/sites/default/files/usp_pdf/EN/gc795.pdf

The Pharmaceutics and Compounding Laboratory, University of North Carolina at Chapel Hill Eshelman School of Pharmacy, 2015. Retrieved from http://pharmlabs.unc.edu/

Community Pharmacy Practice

LAB 28

Preparing and Processing Capsules

■ Introduction

Extemporaneous compounding or *nonsterile compounding* includes preparing capsules. This is a process of combining medication powders with a powder base and filling a blank capsule and may even include additional *fillers* that are used to make up bulk or mask bitter tastes. There are several sizes of capsules, and depending on the final amount of drug in each capsule, the right one must be chosen. For example; if the final amount in milligrams of the capsule being prepared were 800 mg, then the size #000 would be chosen.

When preparing large quantities, a pharmacy will use automated filling machines that can prepare 100 or 200 capsules at one time. For small quantities and for this Lab, you will use the *punch method*. A capsule consists of two parts: the BODY, which is a wider part of the capsule, is punched into the powder; and the CAP, which is the shorter and wider part, is attached to it. Once all the capsules are prepared, a percentage of error formula is calculated to ensure that the weights do not vary more than 90% to 110%, based on guidelines from the United States Pharmacopeia (USP) 795.

> **LAB TIP**
>
> To calculate the error rate, weigh each capsule and then add the weights of each capsule together and divide by the number of capsules. The result has to be in the 90% to 110% range to meet the standards of USP 795.

A *master formula record (FR)* is used as a recipe and includes all the required ingredients and instructions for preparation and documentation. If the compound is written for a specific patient on a prescription, then the directions may vary by physician. In addition to the master FR, a *compounding record (CR)* or *log* will also be generated (on completion of the preparation) to provide a record of the compound itself. This CR will include information such as the prescription number, each ingredient's information, and who made the compound and who checked it.

A *safety data sheet (SDS)* is available for each active ingredient and should be included as part of the documentation for every compound made.

■ Lab Objectives

In this Lab, you will:

- Demonstrate the skills required for interpreting, calculating, and preparing punch method capsules from a prescription.
- Prepare an electronic label from a prescription for a capsule dosage form.
- Complete a repackaging log.
- Identify special requirements for compounded capsules, including the use of equipment, techniques, and patient directions for storage.
- Demonstrate ethics, adhere to patient privacy, and work as a team member in a simulated laboratory scenario.

ASHP goals: 7, 11, 12, 16, 18, 21, 22, 25, 26, 27, 29, 33, 35, 36, 41, and 44.

■ Scenario

In your pharmacy today, you have been assigned to the compounding section. Once calculations are performed and a label is prepared, you must gather the equipment and prepare the capsules. The final product must be recorded, have proper labeling, and be checked at each key interval, as determined by the master FR or recipe.

■ Pre Lab Information

Using the Visual Superscript database, as well as the prescriptions, medications, and supplies provided, review the process for flavoring and reconstituting your prescription. Use a reference source to find storage information (beyond use date [BUD]), and identify any auxiliary labels or special instructions required before entering the prescription.

■ Student Directions

Estimated completion time: 30 minutes

Dr. James Furman
3345 Atrium Drive
Albany, NY 12205
Office: (518) 555-4677
Fax: (518) 555-4679

Date: ___5/20/2017___

Patient Name: ___Samuel Urban___

Address: ___29 Walnut Street, Newton, MA 02456___

℞

Simulated Cafergot 2/100 capsules #10
Take 2 capsules at onset of migraine and at
½-hour intervals until gone.
Refill: ___0___ Do not exceed 8 tablets

DEA: AF5190688

Dr. J. Furman
M.D.

Interpret the above prescription, including all calculations and the days' supply.

Ergotamin/Caffein 2/100 capsules

Interpretation: The patient will take 2 capsules when a headache starts and then a capsule every half hour until the headache is gone or until eight capsules have been taken.

You must make a total of 10 capsules.

 LAB TIP

Use your **master FR** at the end of this Lab to gather the needed ingredients and supplies to prepare this medication.

DD Ergotamine tartarate powder 100 g
DD Powder Caffein anhydrous 100 g
DD SIMBASE POWDER 500 g

STEPS TO PREPARE AND PROCESS CAPSULES

1. Using Lab 22 as a reference, enter the capsules and prepare a prescription for Mr. Urban.

2. After completing the information on the **DRUG AND PACKAGING** form, use the following directions to enter the required ingredients for the capsules.

3. Key in the first few letters of the desired drug ingredient. Select the 0.02 correct drug from the list by clicking on the drug name. Click **OK**.

Search for *DD* for DD Ergotamine tartarate powder.
Select the 100 g for this drug.

LAB TIP

Remember to search using the first two letters of the desired drug, and always review the dose and package size for the item you choose. Once this is done, you will charge for the amount needed to make your compound. In this case, you will need to use 10 mg or 0.01 g; you will charge a total of 0.01 g needed to make the medication.

4. In the *Compound Drug Ingredients* dialog box, type in the correct quantity of drug (in grams) that you will need.

   For this ingredient, you will need 10 mg or 0.01 g (based on calculations performed. The master FR gives the formula for each capsule, and this must be multiplied by 10).

5. Click the **SAVE** 💾 icon on the bottom of the *Compound Drug Ingredients* dialog box.

6. Now, continue to enter the other ingredients from the master formula.

LAB TIP

Remember: The master FR gives the formula for each capsule, and the ingredients all must be multiplied by 10.

7. In the *Compound Drug Ingredients* dialog box, type in the correct quantity of drug (in grams) that you will need.

LAB TIP

If you have more ingredients, add each ingredient one at a time by clicking on the **NEW** 🗋 icon located at the bottom right of the *Drugs* form. Review the steps in this Lab to add each ingredient.

8. Once all of the ingredients are added, click the **CLOSE** ▯ icon on the top right of the toolbar. The compound is now saved.

9. You are now returned to the main screen. Perform a drug look-up procedure to confirm that the new compound has been correctly added to the computer system.

   a. Click on the **DRUG** button on the left side of the screen.

   b. Click the **FIND** 🔍 icon located at the top left of the toolbar.

   c. The *Drug Name Lookup* dialog box appears. Type in the label name of the new compound.
      Enter *ERG/CAF/1/100* for your compound.

   d. Select the correct compound from the list by clicking on the drug name. Click **OK**.

   e. Read through the *Drugs* form to check for accuracy.
      Print the screen, and save it for your instructor.

   f. Click the **CLOSE** ▯ icon on the top right of the toolbar to clear the screen.

STEPS TO PREPARE THE LABEL FOR A COMPOUNDED PRESCRIPTION

1. Once the compound is entered in the database, fill a prescription using the directions in Lab 6 and the **QUICK CODE** you selected for the compound. This will be the prescribed drug for the patient.
   Enter QUICK CODE *EAERG/CAF/1/100*.

Community Pharmacy Practice

2. Type in the appropriate days' supply in the **Prescribed Days Supply** data entry field.

Enter 30 days in the Prescribed Days Supply data entry field.

3. Once the product is compounded, you will need to apply a *Take as Directed* sticker along with the patient label on the container.

STEPS FOR THE PREPARATION OF CAPSULES PROCESS

1. Once the labels are printed, retrieve the ingredients needed from the shelf.

 LAB TIP

Each ingredient has a specific lot number, bar code, and expiration date provided by the U.S. Food and Drug Administration (FDA). To verify that the correct medication is being compounded, this number must match the master FR list of ingredients and the **CR** once finished.

2. Follow the **master FR** provided, and complete each step as it is written.

Master Formula Record
(for training purposes only)

Ergotamine/Caffeine 1/100 capsules
FORMULA: for each capsule

INGREDIENT/DRUG	AMOUNT
DD SIMBASE POWDER	500 g
DD Ergotamine tartarate powder	100 g
DD Powder Caffein anhydrous	100 g

Beyond use date : 180 days

NOTE: This formula is for training purposes only and is not intended for human use. It is recommended that you follow USP <795> recommendations for potency testing which states "each preparation shall contain not less than 90.0% and not more than 110.0% of the theoretically calculated and labeled quantity of active ingredient."

This is for simulation training purposes only and has not been tested in a PCCA lab and all required steps in process should be verified by Instructor.

Suggested Compounding Procedures

1. Wash hands and dress in appropriate protective attire.
2. Assemble ingredients and equipment required for compound.
3. Calculate the amounts needed for each ingredient (must make 10 total capsules).
4. Weigh appropriate amounts of ingredients under observation of RPh.
5. Using the Principles of Geometric Dilution (described below), mix Ergotamin, caffein, and SIMBASE powder together with trituration in a mortar and pestle.
   The particles of powders should be the same throughout and almost appear shiny.
   Principles of Geometric Dilution: This procedure should be followed when mixing an ingredient of a larger quantity with a second (or more) ingredients of a smaller quantity. In this case, the caffein and Ergotamin (active ingredients) are to be mixed into the SIMBASE powder gradually – in small portions. Under no circumstance should the entire quantity of ALL ingredients (powders) be placed in the mortar to start with.
6. Once mixed thoroughly, using the punch method, add powder to the capsule blanks.
7. Assign a BUD after compounding following USP 795 guidelines and complete compounding record/log. Estimated to be 180 days or less.

Warning: *Safety precautions should be taken when compounding and using equipment. Follow all laboratory and product safety guidelines and wear appropriate personal protective equipment.*

---

3. Prepare the **CR** with all required information.

Compounding Record   Drug _____   Date _____

Prescription Number or ID Assigned	Master FR Record # Used	Name and Strength of Compound	Quantity	Actual Net Measurements	Expiration Date	MFG Lot Number	MFG Expiration Date	BUD Assigned	Date Packaged	Tech Initials	RPh Initials

Attach a prescription/patient label if applicable.

ID, Identification; *FR*, formula record; *MFG*, manufacturer; *BUD*, beyond use date; *RPh*, registered pharmacist.

4. Locate the **SDS** for all ingredients using www.pocketnurse.com.

5. Once the pharmacist has completed the verification process, simulate the dispensing to include customer interaction, processing the sale, and final packaging.

RESOURCES

Allen LV, Adejare A, Desselle SP, Felton LA (eds): *Remington: the science and practice of pharmacy*, ed 22, London, 2013, Pharmaceutical Press.

Mosby's drug reference for health professions, ed 4, St Louis, 2014, Mosby.

Pharmaceutical Compounding—Nonsterile Preparations. The United States Pharmacopeial Convention, 2014. Retrieved from http://www.usp.org/sites/default/files/usp_pdf/EN/gc795.pdf

The Pharmaceutics and Compounding Laboratory, University of North Carolina at Chapel Hill, Eshelman School of Pharmacy, 2015. Retrieved from http://pharmlabs.unc.edu/

LAB 29

Preparing and Processing Gels

▪ Introduction

Extemporaneous compounding or *nonsterile compounding* includes preparing gels. A clear, thin, *water-in-oil* (W/O) preparation is formulated to soak into or penetrate the skin. It will have a light, smooth, slightly cool feel, and will typically be compounded by adding powders or solutions to a base and incorporating (mixing) them together with a spatula.

A ***master formula record (FR)*** is used as a recipe and includes all the required ingredients and instructions for preparation and documentation. If the compound is written for a specific patient on a prescription, then the directions may vary by physician. In addition to the master FR, a ***compounding record (CR)*** or ***log*** will also be generated (on completion of the preparation) to provide a record of the compound itself. This CR will include information such as the prescription number, each ingredient's information, and who made the compound and who checked it.

A ***safety data sheet (SDS)*** is available for each active ingredient and should be included as part of the documentation for every compound made.

▪ Lab Objectives

In this Lab, you will:

- Demonstrate the skills required for interpreting, calculating, and preparing a gel compound from a prescription.
- Prepare an electronic label from a prescription for a gel medication.
- Complete a repackaging log.
- Identify special requirements for gel medications, including the use of equipment, techniques, and patient directions for storage.
- Demonstrate ethics, adhere to patient privacy, and work as a team member in a simulated laboratory scenario.

ASHP goals: 7, 11, 12, 16, 18, 21, 22, 25, 26, 27, 29, 33, 35, 36, 41, and 44.

▪ Scenario

In your pharmacy today, you have been assigned to the compounding section. Once calculations are performed and a label is prepared, you must gather the equipment and prepare the gel compound. The final product must be recorded, have proper labeling, and be checked at each key interval, as determined by the **master FR** or recipe.

▪ Pre Lab Information

Using the Visual Superscript database, as well as the prescriptions, medications, and supplies provided, review the process for flavoring and reconstituting your prescription. Use a reference source to find storage information (beyond use date [BUN]), and identify any auxiliary labels or special instructions required before entering the prescription.

Estimated completion time: 30 minutes

Dr. John Smith
739 Stockton Street
Waltham, MA 02454
Office: (339) 333-2121
Fax: (339) 333-2123

Date: _____12/1/2017_____

Patient Name: __Adam Armstrong__

Address: __23 Egmont Street, Waltham, MA 02454__

℞ 5% Simulated Testosterone gel 60 g
Apply bid

Refill: __0__

DEA: AS3456325
State License: 2724141

Dr. J. Smith
M.D.

Interpret the above prescription, including all calculations and the days' supply.

5% Simulated Testosterone gel 60 g

5% is 50 mg per milliliter or gram

$$\frac{50 \text{ mg}}{\text{mL}} = \frac{x}{60 \text{ mL}} = 5 \text{ g}$$

5 g of the powder is needed, and the remainder is 45% of the gel base. Find the difference to get the amount:

60 g – 5 g = 45 g of gel base
Solve for x grams, and you get 45 grams.
You will need 5 g of the DD Powder Testosteron 100 g and 58 g of the DD SIMBASE gel.
DD Powder Testosteron 100 g
DD SIMBASE gel 500 g

 LAB TIP

Use your **master FR** at the end of this Lab to gather the needed ingredients and supplies to prepare this medication.

STEPS TO PREPARE AND PROCESS GELS

1. Using Lab 22 as a reference, enter the compound gel and prepare a prescription for Mr. Armstrong.

2. After completing the information on the **DRUG AND PACKAGING** form, use the following directions to enter the required ingredients for the gel.

3. Key in the first few letters of the desired drug ingredient. Select the correct drug from the list by clicking on the drug name. Click **OK**.

Search *DD* for DD Powder Testosteron 100 g.
Select **100 g** for this drug.

LAB TIP

Remember to search using the first two letters of the desired drug, and always review the dose and package size for the item you choose. Once this is done, you will charge for the amount needed to make your compound.

4. In the *Compound Drug Ingredients* dialog box, type in the correct quantity of drug (in grams) that you will need.

   For this ingredient, you will need 5 g (based on calculations performed).

5. Click the **SAVE** 🖫 icon on the bottom of the *Compound Drug Ingredients* dialog box.

   Enter *Demo Dose SIMBASE* gel 500 g.

6. In the *Compound Drug Ingredients* dialog box, type in the correct quantity of drug (in grams) that you will need.

   You will need to charge for 45 g (based on calculations performed).

 LAB TIP

If you have more ingredients, add each ingredient one at a time by clicking on the **NEW** 🗋 icon located at the bottom right of the *Drugs* form. Review the steps in this Lab to add each ingredient.

7. Once all of the ingredients are added, click the **CLOSE** ▯ icon on the top right of the toolbar. The compound is now saved.

8. You are now returned to the main screen. Perform a drug look-up procedure to confirm that the new compound has been correctly added to the computer system.

   a. Click on the **DRUG** button on the left side of the screen.

   b. Click the **FIND** 🔍 icon located at the top left of the toolbar.

   c. The *Drug Name Lookup* dialog box appears. Type in the label name of the new compound.

      Enter *PATest5%/60g* for your compound.

   d. Select the correct compound from the list by clicking on the drug name. Click **OK**.

   e. Read through the *Drugs* form to check for accuracy.

      Print the screen, and save it for your instructor.

   f. Click the **CLOSE** ▯ icon on the top right of the toolbar to clear the screen.

STEPS TO PREPARE THE LABEL FOR A COMPOUNDED PRESCRIPTION

1. Once the compound is entered in the database, fill a prescription using the directions in Lab 6 and the **QUICK CODE** you selected for the compound. This will be the prescribed drug for the patient.

   Enter QUICK CODE *PATest5%/60g*.

2. Type in the appropriate days' supply in the **PRESCRIBED DAYS SUPPLY** data entry field.

   Enter *30* in the PRESCRIBED DAYS SUPPLY data entry field.

3. Once the product is compounded, you will need to apply a ***For Topical Use Only*** sticker along with the patient label on the container.

1. Once the labels are printed, retrieve the ingredients needed from the shelf.

 LAB TIP

Each ingredient has a specific lot number, bar code, and expiration date provided by the U.S. Food and Drug Administration (FDA). To verify that the correct medication is being compounded, this number must match the master FR list of ingredients and the **CR** once finished.

2. Follow the master FR provided, and complete each step as it is written.

Master Formula Record
(for training purposes only)

Simulated Testosterone 5% Gel 60 g

INGREDIENT/ DRUG	AMOUNT (GM)
DD Testosteron powder	5 g
DD SIMBASE gel 500 G	45 mL

Equipment and Supplies needed

Scale
Spatulas—(2) 6–8in.
Syringe adapter
Weighing boat LG
Alcohol and wipes

Gloves
60 mL syringes (2)
Syringe tip cap
Weighing papers (2 each)

NOTE: It is recommended that you follow USP <795> recommendations for potency testing which states "each preparation shall contain not less than 90.0% and not more than 110.0% of the theoretically calculated and labeled quantity of active ingredient". In order to provide some guidance in this area, use the 'percentage of error" formula to calculate potency if required by Instructor.

This is for simulation training purposes only and has not been tested in a PCCA lab and all required steps in process should be verified by Instructor.

Suggested Compounding Procedures

1. Perform calculations and measure each ingredient separately with a 10% excess (Testosterone on paper) and (SIMBASE in boat).

   NOTE: Some material may be lost due to sticking to sides or container. Making 10% more will provide enough to measure the full 30g needed.
2. Have your Instructor check weights of each.
3. Using the spatula, place the SIMBASE gel and Testosterone in a glass mortar.
4. Using geometric dilution, gradually add powder to base and mix thoroughly. Combine the two ingredients completely.
5. Once mixed, draw up all the preparation into the 60ml syringe.
6. Connect the other syringe to the end by using the syringe connector and transfer contents back and forth continuing to mix.
7. Once mixed, add the syringe tip securely.
8. Assign a BUD after compounding following USP <795> guidelines and complete compounding record/log. Estimated to be 30 days or less.

Warning: *Safety precautions should be taken when compounding and using equipment. Follow all laboratory and product safety guidelines and wear appropriate personal protective equipment.*

3. Prepare the **CR** with all required information.

Compounding Record Drug _____ Date _____

Prescription Number or ID Assigned	Master FR Record # Used	Name and Strength of Compound	Quantity	Actual Net Measurements	Expiration Date	MFG Lot Number	MFG Expiration Date	BUD Assigned	Date Packaged	Tech Initials	RPh Initials

Attach a prescription/patient label if applicable.
ID, Identification; *FR,* formula record; *MFG,* manufacturer; *BUD,* beyond use date; *RPh,* registered pharmacist.

4. Locate the **SDS** for all ingredients using www.pocketnurse.com.

5. Once the pharmacist has completed the verification process, simulate the dispensing to include customer interaction, processing the sale, and final packaging.

RESOURCES

Allen LV, Adejare A, Desselle SP, Felton LA (eds): *Remington: the science and practice of pharmacy,* ed 22, London, 2013, Pharmaceutical Press.

Mosby's drug reference for health professions, ed 4, St Louis, 2014, Mosby.

Pharmaceutical Compounding—Nonsterile Preparations. The United States Pharmacopeial Convention, 2014. Retrieved from http://www.usp.org/sites/default/files/usp_pdf/EN/gc795.pdf

The Pharmaceutics and Compounding Laboratory, University of North Carolina at Chapel Hill, Eshelman School of Pharmacy, 2015. Retrieved from http://pharmlabs.unc.edu/

Pulling the Pieces Together (Community Pharmacy Practice)

The Pharmacy Management Software manual is separated into pharmacy practice sections and is designed to teach the functions of automated simulation software by using detailed specific or isolated Lab exercises. Technicians in community practice work directly with customers, physicians, and outside (third-party) payers daily, and tasks performed include:

- Data entry and maintenance of electronic patient profiles
- Medication review information (Medication Therapy Management [MTM])
- Inventory control and insurance
- Reporting, returns, and recalls
- Controlled substances
- Nonsterile compounding
- All forms of medication preparation and distribution
- Wellness information, over-the-counter (OTC) medications, nondurable medical equipment, and durable medical equipment (DME) items

Individually working through each task, starting with computer data entry and completing preparation of the medication with a prepared Lab exercise and a list of suggested supplies (found in the Instructor Manual), allows skills to be practiced in a simulated community or retail laboratory setting.

Once the Lab exercises are completed, the program becomes the database label program to be used throughout the entire program for community exercises. In conjunction with the proper equipment and supplies, this program allows the trainee to complete and retain documentation of community practice skills needed before entering the pharmacy workforce.

Community Pharmacy Practice (Comprehensive Exercises)

▪ Introduction

The Pharmacy Management Software manual is separated into pharmacy practice sections and is designed to teach the functions of automated simulation software by using detailed specific or isolated Lab exercises. Technicians in community practice work directly with customers, physicians, and outside (third-party) payers daily.

Beginning early in a pharmacy program, the student will complete each Lab in sequence to learn all the skills associated with day-to-day activities in the community setting. Individually working through each task, starting with computer data entry and completing the preparation of the medication with a prepared Lab exercise and a list of suggested supplies (found in the Instructor Manual), allows skills to be practiced as isolated and sequential exercises in a simulated community or retail laboratory setting. The form provided, once signed by all parties, is kept with supporting documentation for the student files.

Now that individual Lab exercises are completed, the form can be used as a final review of sequential exercises. Putting it all together in scenarios and team activities using a simulated community Lab will reinforce each skill and task and show the student how the community practice environment works. The program has now become the label and database system for the mock pharmacy setting, and prescriptions provided in this section can be assigned. In addition, the database label program is used throughout the entire program for community exercises.

In conjunction with the proper equipment and supplies, the program allows the trainee to complete and retain documentation of community practice skills needed before entering the pharmacy workforce.

▪ Lab Objectives

In this Lab, you will:

- Use the skills learned to perform necessary computer functions to enter a new prescription into a pharmacy system and process it for customer pickup.
- Use the skills learned to process refills for customer pickup.
- Use the knowledge gained to simulate real tasks such as prior approvals, refill authorization, billing, and verification of correct patient and medications that are performed in a community setting.

▪ Student Directions

Estimated completion time: 120 minutes

1. Use the prescriptions provided in this Lab to simulate the processes of preparing medications for customers.
2. Interpret the new prescriptions, input the data, and prepare labels, as well as perform adjudication for insurance and process cash transactions.
3. Refills should be processed from the list of calls received from the patients.
4. Once completed, assemble the stock bottle, the prepared medication, the original prescription (if applicable), and any other documentation required for verification by your instructor.

Dr. Ramon Ramirez
134 Boylston Street
Cambridge, MA 02139
Office: (617) 479-3400
Fax: (617) 479-3402

Date: _____11/1/2017_____

Patient Name: ___Fredonna Clift___

Address: ___222 Mason Street, Cambridge, MA___

R͏x

Lasix 20 mg #30
1 daily prn for edema

Refill: ___1___

DEA: AR3587726

Dr. R. Ramirez
M.D.

Dr. Jasmine Abbosh
836 Farmington Avenue
Worcester, MA 01601
Office: (617) 232-9911
Fax: (617) 734-6340

Date: _____11/27/2017_____

Patient Name: ___Mary Horton___

Address: ___9788 Florence Street, Worchester, MA___

R͏x

NTG 1/150 g
1 tab SL chest pain #100
Lisinopril 10 mg 1 tab po qd #30

Refill: ___2___

DEA: BA4884533

Dr. J. Abbosh
M.D.

Dr. Jasmine Abbosh
836 Farmington Avenue
Worcester, MA 01601
Office: (617) 232-9911
Fax: (617) 734-6340

Date: _3/23/2017_

Patient Name: _Ernest Hatcher_

Address: _4546 Maywood Street, Worchester, MA_

Rx

Ventolin #2 MDI 2 puffs q 3-4 hrs prn
Zyrtex 10 mg 1 qd #30

Refill: _0_

DEA: BA4884533

Dr. J. Abbosh

M.D.

Dr. Jasmine Abbosh
836 Farmington Avenue
Worcester, MA 01601
Office: (617) 232-9911
Fax: (617) 734-6340

Date: _3/21/2017_

Patient Name: _Floyd Ellis_

Address: _73 Birch Street, Worchester, MA_

Rx

Glucophage 500 mg ÷ qd #30
Folic Acid ÷ mg #30
Inderal 40 mg ÷ bid #60
Zyloprin 300 mg ÷ qd #30

Refill: _4_

DEA: BA4884533

Dr. J. Abbosh

M.D.

Dr. Samuel Adams
1234 Walnut Street
Allston, MA 02134
Office: (617) 387-4500
Fax: (617) 387-4502

Date: _____1/4/2017_____

Patient Name: ___Floyd Ellis___

Address: ___5489 Pratt Street, Allston, MA___

R͟x

*Albuterol sulf 0.083% (2.5 mg/3 mL)
2.5 mg q 3 doses, then 5 mg q 4 hrs prn
via nebulizer*

Refill: ___0___

DEA: AA4562131

Dr. S. Adams
M.D.

Dr. Joseph Gaffney
5575 Vine Street
Margate City, NY 04082
Office: (609) 555-6671
Fax: 609) 555-6673

Date: _____12/24/2017_____

Patient Name: ___Douglas Richards___

Address: ___844 South Union Avenue, Margate City, NY___

R͟x

*Prilosec 30 mg 1 cap qd #30
Ambien 5 mg prn for sleep #15
Flomax 0.4 mg qd with meal #30*

Refill: ___0___

DEA: BG2019734

Dr. J. Gaffney
M.D.

Dr. Joseph Gaffney
5575 Vine Street
Margate City, NY 04082
Office: (609) 555-6671
Fax: (609) 555-6673

Date: _____ 2/16/2017 _____

Patient Name: ___Natasha Romanov___

Address: ___62 Amherst Avenue, Margate City, NY___

R℞

Adderall XR 1 qd #30

Refill: ___0___

DEA: BG2019734

Dr. J. Gaffney
M.D.

Dr. Harold Wilson
901 Kent Street
Allston, MA 02134
Office: (617) 555-9900
Fax: (617) 555-9902

Date: _____ 11/24/2017 _____

Patient Name: ___Harry Zinn___

Address: ___3331 Everett Street, Allston, MO___

R℞

NTG 2% ointment
Apply 15 mg (1 in) q 8 hrs

Refill: ___0___

DEA: AW7776668

Dr. H. Wilson
M.D.

Dr. Harold Wilson
901 Kent Street
Allston, MA 02134
(617) 555-9900
Fax: (617) 555-9902

Date: _____3/4/2017_____

Patient Name: ___Mrytle York_____

Address: ___98805 Royal Street, Allston, MA_____

Rx

Nystatin susp 5 mL po qid
S/S x 10 days

Refill: ___1___

DEA: AW7776668

Dr. H. Wilson
M.D.

Dr. Harold Wilson
901 Kent Street
Allston, MA 02134
Office: (617) 555-9900
Fax: (617) 555-9902

Date: _____6/6/2017_____

Patient Name: ___Charles Yost_____

Address: ___88 Easton Street, Allston, MA_____

Rx

Keflex 500 mg
1 tab q 6 hrs x 10 days
Lidocaine viscous S/S i tsp #C

Refill: ___0___

DEA: AW7776668

Dr. H. Wilson
M.D.

Dr. James Unger
730 Beacon Street
Newton, MA 02456
Office: (617) 443-6677
Fax: (617) 443-6679

Date: _____5/31/2017_____

Patient Name: ___Dorothy Zucker_____

Address: ___3201 Chestnut Street, Newton, MA_____

℞

Vistaril 25 mg
qid prn for anxiety #XXX
Metformin 500 mg tid ac #90

Refill: ___0___

DEA: AU6624438

Dr. J. Unger
M.D.

Dr. Kerry Alexander
355 Seneca Drive
Cold Spring, NY 10516
Office: (845) 555-1234
Fax: (845) 555-1236

Date: _____10/30/2017_____

Patient Name: ___Sean Finnegan_____

Address: ___17 Garden Street, Cold Spring, NY_____

℞

Donnatal liquid
5-10 mL with 30 mL Maalox prn
Disp: 8 oz

Refill: ___1___

DEA: AA4153754

Dr. K. Alexander
M.D.

Dr. Kerry Alexander
355 Seneca Drive
Cold Spring, NY 10516
Office: (845) 555-1234
Fax: (845) 555-1236

Date: _____3/17/2017_____

Patient Name: _____Sean Finnegan_____

Address: _____17 Garden Street, Cold Spring, NY_____

℞

Refill: ___3___

Timoptic 1/2% #1 bottle
1 gtt ou bid
Synthroid 50 mcg 1 po qd

DEA: AA4153754

Dr. K. Alexander
M.D.

Dr. Kerry Alexander
355 Seneca Drive
Cold Spring, NY 10516
Office: (845) 555-1234
Fax: (845) 555-1236

Date: _____10/25/2017_____

Patient Name: _____Bernice Good_____

Address: _____90 Whitehill Place, Cold Spring, NY_____

℞

Refill: ___3___

Prednisone 200 mg/day x 7 days,
then 100 mg every other day. Disp: x 1 month
Alprazolam 0.1 mg tid prn anxiety #50

DEA: AA4153754

Dr. K. Alexander
M.D.

Section II

Institutional Pharmacy Practice

INTRODUCTION TO THE WORKFLOW OF INSTITUTIONAL PHARMACY PRACTICE

Institutional pharmacy practice includes pharmacies that dispense medications to patients who are considered inpatient. These patients may require assistance with taking their medications and can include unique packaging and medication delivery to a home or facility. The technician's role consists of working directly with pharmacy personnel and other health care professionals in other departments, data entry, and inventory control using automation, pharmacology, laws and regulations, and record keeping. The facility may be in a hospital, home health (long-term care [LTC]), hospice, rehabilitation or subacute facility, or clinic. Each state has specific rules and ratios, but the technician works directly with the patients and pharmacists every day.

The Lab exercises in this section provide detailed steps to teach and use the Visual SuperScript software applications for entering physician orders and maintaining and editing patient information in the electronic profile, with all of the aspects of physician order processing from interpretation to a finished product.

The workflow for institutional practice starts with the physician order. By simulating each function in isolation and then combining the sequences as team members or with partners, the workflow allows real-world practice in the laboratory setting before the pharmacy technician enters the externship phase of training.

Sterile or aseptic (intravenous [IV]) preparations, bulk repackaging or 30-day cards with automation, and inventory of emergency medications are also common tasks performed by technicians in an institutional setting and are included in this section. In addition, Labs in this section include the label and data entry process for common hospitalized patients, profile management and LTC medications, and include the hands-on exercises to create each form using simulated medications.

LAB 30

Medication Recalls, Inventory Returns, and Disposal Considerations

■ Introduction

When working in pharmacy, you will need to manage the daily tasks with inventory control, which will include ordering and identifying medications that should be pulled from current stock because of overstock, expiration, recalls, or destruction (controlled substances). Each medication has a specific National Drug Code (NDC) number and, if recalled by U.S. Food and Drug Administration (FDA) or the manufacturer, this NDC number will be used as an identifier along with the lot number and the manufacturer's expiration date. The database will also use this information to identify current stock and can be reviewed through the **Drug** tab feature on the right.

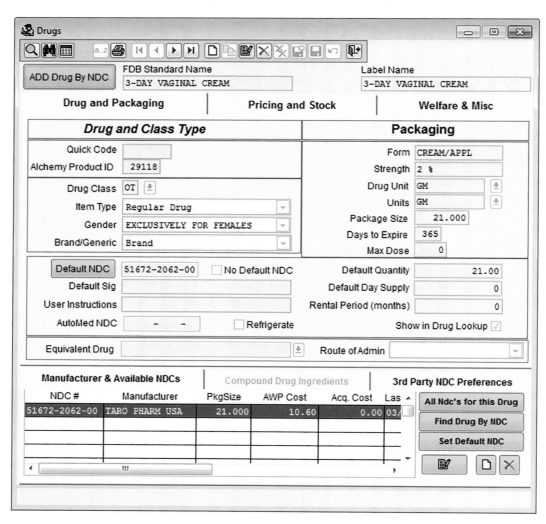

In most cases, wholesalers will allow a return if a medication is short dated or damaged. Returning a medication requires the inventory to be depleted in the database system and then the old stock pulled from the shelf. Some companies' sole job is to process returns for those medications that cannot be returned to the manufacturers. An example of a nonreturnable medication would be amoxicillin suspension once it is mixed or a compounded medication such as an ointment or cream. Once the old stock is removed from the database, new inventory can be ordered and, following Lab 5 directions, added to the system.

An example of a recall follows. The drug being recalled is sodium bicarbonate injection. The identifiers include the NDC number, lot number, and manufacturer's expiration date.

Hospira Issues a Voluntary Recall for One Lot of Sodium Bicarbonate Injection, USP Due to the Presence of a Particulate

FOR IMMEDIATE RELEASE
March 18, 2016

CONTACT	Consumers	Media
	1-888-345-4680	610-329-1340

ANNOUNCEMENT

LAKE FOREST, Ill. – Hospira, Inc., a Pfizer company, is voluntarily recalling one lot of 8.4% Sodium Bicarbonate Injection, USP (NDC: 0409-6625-02, Lot 56-148-EV, Expiry 1AUG2017) at the hospital/retail level due to the presence of a particulate within a single–dose glass fliptop vial. The issue was identified through a confirmed complaint.

If the particulate is not observed prior to IV administration and breaks off into smaller particulates, passing through the catheter, it may result in localized inflammation, allergic reaction, including anaphylaxis, granuloma formation or microembolic effects (IV only). Larger particulates may block the infusion of solution, potentially resulting in a delay in therapy. The likelihood of risk to the patient is low due to the high detectability of the particulate prior to or at the point of care. Although serious in nature, the probability of harm in this case is low due to the high detectability of the non-conformance.

To date, Hospira has not received reports of any adverse events associated with this issue for this lot. Hospira places the utmost emphasis on patient safety and product quality at every step in the manufacturing and supply chain process.

The product is packaged 50 mEq (1mEq/mL), 4.2 grams (84 mg/mL), 50mL, Single-dose, packaged 4 boxes of 25 vials per case. The lot was distributed nationwide in the U.S. to wholesalers and hospitals in December 2015. Hospira has initiated an investigation to determine the root cause and corrective and preventive actions.

Sodium Bicarbonate Injection, USP is indicated in the treatment of metabolic acidosis; in the treatment of certain drug intoxications, in poisoning by salicylates or methyl alcohol and in certain hemolytic reactions. Sodium bicarbonate also is indicated in severe diarrhea, which is often accompanied by significant loss of bicarbonate.

Anyone with an existing inventory of the recalled lot should stop use and distribution and quarantine the product immediately. Inform Healthcare Professionals in your organization of this recall. If you have further distributed the recalled product, please notify any accounts or additional locations which may have received the recalled product from you. Further, please instruct entities that may have received the recalled product from you that if they redistributed the product, they should notify their accounts, locations or facilities of the recall to the hospital/retail level. Hospira will be notifying its direct customers via a recall letter and is arranging for impacted product to be returned to Stericycle in the United States. For additional assistance, call Stericycle at 1-888-965-6077 between the hours of 8 a.m. to 5 p.m. ET, Monday through Friday. For clinical inquiries, please contact Hospira using the information provided below.

Hospira Contact	Contact Information	Areas of Support
Hospira Global Complaint Management	1-800-441-4100 (8am-5pm CT, M-F) (ProductComplaintsPP@hospira.com)	To report adverse events or product complaints
Hospira Medical Communications	1-800-615-0187 or medcom@hospira.com (Available 24 hours a day/7 days per week)	Medical inquiries

Adverse reactions or quality problems experienced with the use of this product may be reported to the FDA's MedWatch Adverse Event Reporting program either online, by regular mail or by fax.

- Complete and submit the report Online: www.fda.gov/medwatch/report.htm
- Regular Mail or Fax: Download form www.fda.gov/MedWatch/getforms.htm or call 1-800-332-1088 to request a reporting form, then complete and return to the address on the pre-addressed form, or submit by fax to 1-800-FDA-0178

This recall is being executed with the knowledge of the U.S. Food and Drug Administration.

From the U.S. Food and Drug Administration. Accessed March 30, 2016, http://www.fda.gov/Safety/Recalls/ucm491476.htm.

MEDICATION SAFETY CONSIDERATION

Entering the correct data when choosing a particular medication for dispensing is extremely important, because the *drug database* will provide a description of the drug and include the NDC number, manufacturer, package size, and cost.

■ Lab Objectives

In this Lab, you will:

- Perform the task of searching the database for a medication that has been recalled or requires removal for destruction attributable to expiration.
- Remove the assigned medication, and prepare reverse distributor documentation.
- Demonstrate the steps required to identify the safety data sheet (SDS) for a chosen medication, and add notes to the database reflecting changes.
- Verify each other's work (simulate *tech-check-tech*) when performing a recall exercise.

■ Scenario

Today, you are working in a simulated retail setting and learning how to perform inventory functions for recalls, returns, and identification of SDSs and medications in stock.

■ Pre Lab Information

The Lab exercise will teach you how to perform the steps of using the drug database to find a recently recalled medication and any medication scheduled for destruction because of expiration. Once you identify the inventory in the database, notes will be added to document the removal and preparation of the medication for return to a destruction company. Working with a partner (classmate) will simulate the activity in a typical hospital or community environment.

■ Student Directions

Estimated completion time: 30 minutes

1. Read through the steps in the Lab before performing the Lab exercise.
2. After reading through the Lab, perform the required steps to enter provider information.
3. Complete the exercise at the end of the Lab.

STEPS TO VERIFY AND REMOVE CURRENT DRUG INVENTORY

You have learned how to add new drugs to the software database, as well as change the order amount. Now, if a medication needs to be removed from inventory, then the following steps will guide you to find a drug by its NDC number and adjust its current quantities to zero (0).

1. Access the main screen of Visual SuperScript.

2. Click on the **DRUG** button located on the left side of the screen. The *Drugs* dialog box will appear.

3. Click on the **FIND** [Q] icon at the top left of the *Drugs* dialog box.

4. Type in the first three letters of the drug to search, and click **OK** to select the correct drug and dosage.

> Type *SOD* for sodium bicarbonate 8.4% 50 mL vial.

5. In the field next to the **DEFAULT NDC** button, you will find the current NDC number for stock on the shelf.

6. If the NDC number matches the stock, then the current stock should be removed from inventory (database) and from the shelf.

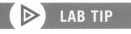

LAB TIP

Use the manufacturer and available NDC numbers to identify other options for manufacturers' recall information to identify current stock levels with appropriate NDC numbers listed.

7. Choose the **Pricing and Stock** tab at the top of the screen.

8. If there is current inventory, click on the **Add/Adjust Stock** button.

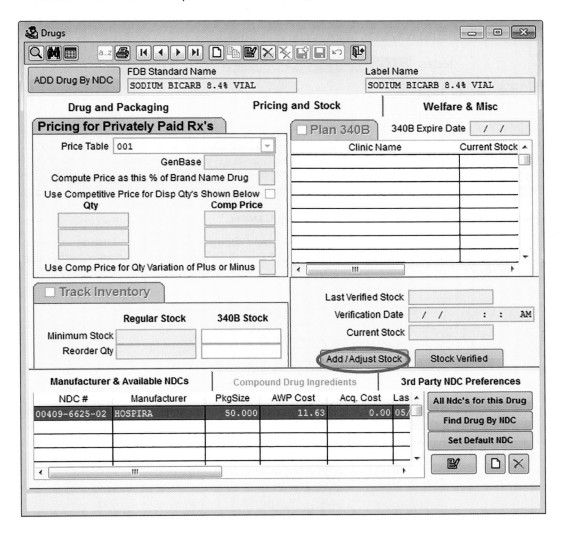

9. The *Drug Stock* dialog box appears. Type quantity to **0**.

10. Type the lot number as ***56148EV*** as seen on the FDA recall in this Lab.

11. Type expiration date ***8/17*** as seen on the recall information from the FDA.

12. In the *Notes* field, add the following notation, along with the current date.

All removed for a recall.

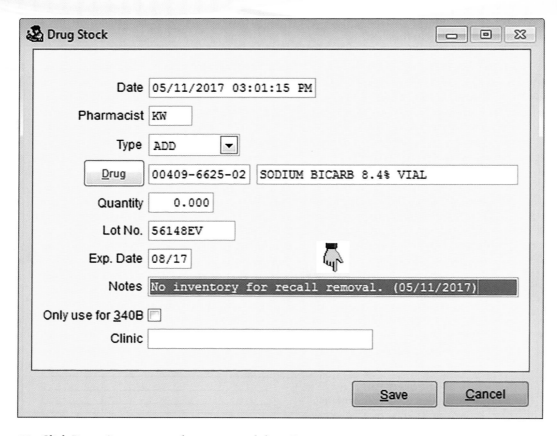

13. Click **Prnt Scrn** to save the screen, and then **Cancel**.

Note: This is a simulated exercise to demonstrate the process used for adjusting inventory. If inventory did exist for this drug, you would save these changes before closing, rather than canceling.

U. S. DEPARTMENT OF JUSTICE – DRUG ENFORCEMENT ADMINISTRATION
REGISTRANT RECORD OF CONTROLLED SUBSTANCES DESTROYED
FORM DEA-41

A. REGISTRANT INFORMATION

Registered Name:	DEA Registration Number:
Registered Address:	
City: State:	Zip Code:
Telephone Number:	Contact Name:

B. ITEM DESTROYED
1. Inventory

	National Drug Code or DEA Controlled Substances Code Number	Batch Number	Name of Substance	Strength	Form	Pkg. Qty.	Number of Full Pkgs.	Partial Pkg. Count	Total Destroyed
Examples	16590-598-60	N/A	Kadian	60mg	Capsules	60	2	0	120 Capsules
	0555-0767-02	N/A	Adderall	5mg	Tablet	100	0	83	83 Tablets
	9050	B02120312	Codeine	N/A	Bulk	1.25 kg	N/A	N/A	1.25 kg
1.									
2.									
3.									
4.									
5.									
6.									
7.									

2. Collected Substances

	Returned Mail-Back Package	Sealed Inner Liner	Unique Identification Number	Size of Sealed Inner Liner	Quantity of Packages(s)/Liner(s) Destroyed
Examples	X		MBP1106, MBP1108 - MBP1110, MBP112	N/A	5
		X	CRL1007 - CRL1027	15 gallon	21
		X	CRL1201	5 gallon	1
1.					
2.					
3.					
4.					
5.					
6.					
7.					

Form DEA-41　　　　　　*See instructions on reverse (page 2) of form.*

Courtesy Drug Enforcement Administration, Washington, DC.

Institutional Pharmacy Practice

DEA-41 Pg. 2

C. METHOD OF DESTRUCTION

Date of Destruction:	Method of Destruction:
Location or Business Name:	
Address:	

City:	State:	Zip Code:

D. WITNESSES

I declare under penalty of perjury, pursuant to 18 U.S.C. 1001, that I personally witnessed the destruction of the above-described controlled substances to a non-retrievable state and that all of the above is true and correct.

Printed name of first authorized employee witness:	Signature of first witness:	Date:
Printed name of second authorized employee witness:	Signature of second witness:	Date:

E. INSTRUCTIONS

1. <u>Section A. REGISTRANT INFORMATION</u>: The registrant destroying the controlled substance(s) shall provide their DEA registration number and the name and address indicated on their valid DEA registration, in addition to a current telephone number and a contact name, if different from the name on the valid DEA registration.

2. <u>Section B. (1) Inventory</u>: This part shall be used by registrants destroying lawfully possessed controlled substances, other than those described in Section B(2). In each row, indicate the National Drug Code (NDC) for the controlled substance destroyed, or if the substance has no NDC, indicate the DEA Controlled Substances Code Number for the substance; if the substance destroyed is in bulk form, indicate the batch number, if available. In each row, indicate the name, strength, and form of the controlled substance destroyed, and the number of capsules, tablets, etc., that are in a full package (pkg. qty.). If destroying the full quantity of the controlled substance, indicate the number of packages destroyed (number of full pkgs.). If destroying a partial package, indicate the partial count of the capsules, tablets, etc. destroyed (partial pkg. count). If destroying a controlled substance in bulk form, indicate that the substance is in bulk form (form) and the weight of the substance destroyed (pkg. qty.). In each row, indicate the total number of each controlled substance destroyed (total destroyed).

3. <u>Section B. (2) Collected Substances</u>: This part shall be used by registrants destroying controlled substances obtained through an authorized collection activity in accordance with 21 U.S.C. 822(g). In each row, indicate whether registrant is destroying a mail-back package or an inner liner. If destroying a mail-back package, enter each unique identification number separated by a comma and/or as a list in a sequential range and total quantity of packages being destroyed. If destroying an inner liner, enter each unique identification number separated by a comma and/or as a list in a sequential range based on the size of the liners destroyed and the total quantity of inner liners being destroyed. In the case of mail-back packages or inner liners received from a law enforcement agency which do not have a unique identification number or clearly marked size, include the name of the law enforcement agency and, if known, the size of the inner liner or package. DO NOT OPEN ANY MAIL-BACK PACKAGE OR INNER LINER; AN INVENTORY OF THE CONTENTS OF THE PACKAGES OR LINERS IS PROHIBITED BY LAW AND IS NOT REQUIRED BY THIS FORM.

4. If additional space is needed for items destroyed in Section B, attach to this form additional page(s) containing the requested information for each controlled substance destroyed.

5. <u>Section C. METHOD OF DESTRUCTION</u>: Provide the date, location, and method of destruction. The method of destruction must render the controlled substance to a state of non-retrievable and meet all applicable destruction requirements.

6. <u>Section D. WITNESSES</u>: Two authorized employees must declare by signature, under penalty of perjury, that such employees personally witnessed the destruction of the controlled substances listed in Section B in the manner described in Section C.

7. You are not required to submit this form to DEA, unless requested to do so. This form must be kept as a record of destruction and be available by the registrant for at least two years in accordance with 21 U.S.C. 827.

ADDITIONAL EXERCISES

The following medications have been identified as expired or overstocked and should be pulled for return to the wholesaler. Use the steps as outlined in this Lab to check inventory for any current stock.

Perform the *Look-Up* procedure for each drug listed, and determine whether any current inventory matches these drugs in the database. Identify how many medications are currently in stock under the **Pricing and Stock** tab.

DRUG	NATIONAL DRUG CODE	CURRENT INVENTORY
Furosemide 40 mg	00172-2907-10	
Lasix 40 mg tablet	0039-0050-10	
Singulair 4 mg chew tab	0006-0711-28	
Prozac weekly 90 mg cap	0002-3004-75	
Diflorasone 0.05% cream 60 g	0002-3004-75	

LAB 31

Repackaging Medications for an Automated Dispensing Cabinet Using Bar Coding Technology

■ Introduction

In recent pharmacy practice settings, there has been a push to automate the dispensing process for both speed and accuracy. Information systems use a bar coding verification process to ensure the right medication is being processed by using the National Drug Code (NDC), lot number, and expiration date.

New systems, such as computerized prescription order entry (CPOE), and e-prescribing, take out the handwriting interpretation factor, which accounts for many errors in the process. CPOE also aids in the inventory and billing process; patients are electronically charged or credited in real time when using medications from automated cabinets. However, this process is still not 100% error free and requires a technician to use the knowledge and skills in which they have been trained.

An automated dispensing cabinet (ADC) is the best way to make medications available for the patients at the nurses' level. The cabinet can stock many medications, and using a CPOE system, the pharmacist enters the patient order, and the nurse can pull the medication for dispensing for each specific patient. The verification process can include arm-band scanners, and inventory control uses the CPOE system as well. Pockets are assigned at the pharmacy main cabinet, and technicians fill or refill the cabinet using the electronic bar coding verification system.

Medications in the cabinet are in single or UNIT dose form. Using stock bottles to prepare labels and single doses for medications is a daily activity for the pharmacy technician. Repackaging uses the information from the stock bottle and assigns a beyond use date (BUD), which is usually a year, for the unit dose (UD) packages being prepared. These medications are then LOADED into each cabinet on the floors.

MEDICATION SAFETY CONSIDERATION

The National Coordinating Council for Medication Error Reporting and Prevention (NCC MERP) was established by the United States Pharmacopeia (USP) to address error-prevention strategies and prevention.

■ Lab Objectives

In this Lab, you will:

- Learn how to verify medications for repackaging by scanning stock bottles using bar code technology or NDC verification through the **DAILY ACTIVITY LOG** window.
- Learn how to repackage bulk medications for ADC stock filling.

■ Scenario

You are working in a hospital today in the ADC area. Some medications need to be repackaged in single units for the floor dispensing units. You will use a bar code scanner or manual verification to prepare labels and medication in unit-dose packaging.

■ Pre Lab Information

Prepare a compound for each medication listed, and repackage in unit-dose packaging for distribution in the ADC area. Once checked by the pharmacist (instructor), add these to the cabinet in the lab for inventory. You will use gloves and place medications in each pocket and then apply labels printed from the software. For the liquid medications, you will use the oral syringes and caps provided.

MEDICATION SAFETY CONSIDERATION

The Institute for Safe Medication Practices (ISMP) publishes several lists to aid in error prevention such as **High Alert**, **TALL Man Lettering**, and **Do Not Crush** drugs, which can be found by visiting the ISMP Web site (http://www.ismp.org/).

■ Student Directions

Estimated completion time: 30 minutes

1. Read through the steps in the Lab before performing the Lab exercise.
2. After reading through the Lab, perform the required steps to complete the tasks in each scenario.

ENTER A NEW INTRAVENOUS MEDICATION (DRUG)

1. Check your printer settings.

2. Go to **OPTIONS** on the top toolbar of Visual Superscript.

3. Choose **RX LABEL OPTIONS**.

4. Change *Label Type* to LM32.

5. *Workflow Label* can remain as the default—LM32.

6. Click the **SAVE** 💾 icon at the bottom right of the window.

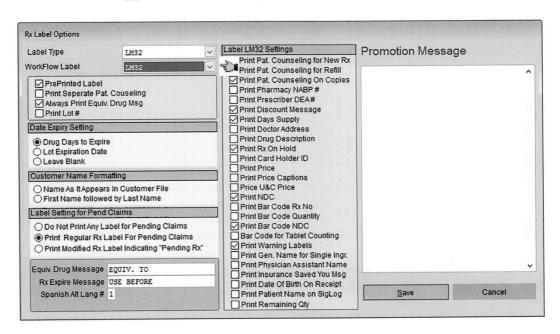

STEPS TO PREPARE THE LABELS FROM BULK BOTTLES

1. Access the main screen of Visual SuperScript.

2. Verify the NDC, lot number, and expiration date on the bulk bottle.
   List of medications to be prepared:
   - Benadryl 12.5 mg/5 mL oral liquid—prepare 10 syringes
   - Metformin 500 tablets—prepare 50 units

3. The software will require a BUD in most cases. *If a BUD is not automatically assigned at 1 year for oral tablets or less for the bulk bottle date, then manually assign the date. For oral liquids, assign the date as 6 months or less if the bulk bottle is less.*

4. Prepare 50 count of the oral tablets and 10 each for the oral liquid syringes.

5. Enter each medication compound following the steps in Lab 22 for extemporaneous compounding.

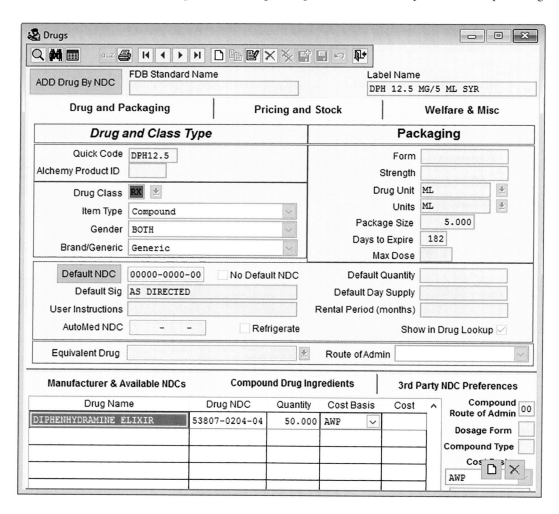

 LAB TIP

Compounding does not require more than one ingredient to be mixed. If medication is removed from its original manufacturer's package and placed in unit dose packaging, it is considered compounding.

6. Repeat the process for all drugs. Verify with the patient (your fellow student) that all information is current in the *Drugs* dialog box. Use the **Prnt Scrn** function to print a copy for each medication for your instructor to review.

STEPS TO PREPARE MEDICATIONS IN UNIT DOSE FORM

1. Once the labels for both medications are verified, ONE AT A TIME, place the medication in either a pocket or syringe pocket and add labels. Keep the stock bottles with each medication prepared for verification by the instructor. If the medication you are preparing is included in the ISMP listing for high alert or TALL man lettering, then type the label name(s) to reflect this. Visit the Web site provided in the previous **Medication Safety Consideration** box to access the listings.

   For example: Diphenhydramine should be typed on the labels as *diphenhydrAMINE*.

2. Once checked, add these medications to the ADC inventory per the cabinet instructions.

MEDICATION SAFETY CONSIDERATION

Prepare only one medication at a time, and separate each medication once it is ready for checking. This process will keep you from mixing up medications in the UD packages; some liquids or tablets may be the same color and shape.

Institutional Pharmacy Practice

LAB 32

Medication Reconciliation

■ Introduction

Preventing medication errors combines many strategies to keep patients from harm, including automation, training and education, and a commitment to excellence. The Institute for Healthcare Improvement (IHI) is an organization that uses medication reconciliation as a process of recording and reviewing a complete list of medications for a patient. Technicians participate in this process by entering information into a database and creating an electronic profile that can then be reviewed by the physician, pharmacist, patient, and other providers.

As the patient moves from one facility or pharmacy or from one caregiver to another, the profile should be updated to provide the most current list of medications.

MEDICATION SAFETY CONSIDERATION

Remember: Patient profiles are only as complete as you make them, and using the ability to add notes and over-the-counter medications (OTC), vitamins, herbals, and durable and nondurable products, such as insulin needles or lancets, is the best practice for creating a complete patient history. All medications, including those not actually dispensed at your pharmacy, should be included in the profile to ensure that the medication reconciliation report information will be as accurate as possible.

■ Lab Objectives

In this Lab, you will:

- Look up patient profiles, and complete inpatient and outpatient medication reconciliation forms for a patient. The outpatient form will be used to take to a new physician appointment (specialist). The inpatient form will be used when a patient is being discharged from the hospital and is entering a rehabilitation center.
- Edit and enter information into the database to update the patient profiles.
- Demonstrate the ability to perform the tasks a technician should complete for data entry if a patient provides information for a new allergy.

■ Scenario

You will continue to work together in the simulated laboratory by adding the function of reviewing and preparing a complete profile, which will require some profile data entry and adding notes. You may refer to previous Labs.

■ Pre Lab Information

You have learned all the steps of data entry and of maintaining a patient profile in a community and institutional setting from previous Labs. Now, you will add the additional practice of reviewing and recording the data found in a profile for a requested patient medication reconciliation report.

■ Student Directions

Estimated completion time: 30 minutes

1. Read through the steps in the Lab before performing the Lab exercise.
2. After reading through the Lab, perform the required steps to create the medication reconciliation form for each patient.
3. Complete the exercise at the end of the Lab.

STEPS TO ADDING AND EDITING INFORMATION TO A PATIENT'S PROFILE AND COMPLETING A MEDICATION RECONCILIATION REPORT

1. Access the main screen of Visual SuperScript.

2. Click on **FILL Rx's** located on the left side of the menu screen. The *Prescription Processing* form appears.

3. Click on the **CUS HISTORY/REFILL** icon on the left of the *Prescription Processing* form to access complete lists of medications for a given patient.

4. You will then be prompted to the *Customer* data entry field (highlighted in blue). Type the first three letters of the last name and hit **ENTER**.

Type *ENG* for English, Brooke.
Validate the date of birth (DOB): 8.10.64

5. Select the appropriate customer by double-clicking on the customer name or by clicking **OK**.

   Note: The customer's profile with all medications that have been entered into the database will be listed.

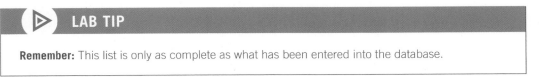

LAB TIP

Remember: This list is only as complete as what has been entered into the database.

6. Verify with the patient (your fellow student) that all medications are current in the profile. Use the **PRNT SCRN** function to share this with the patient for review.

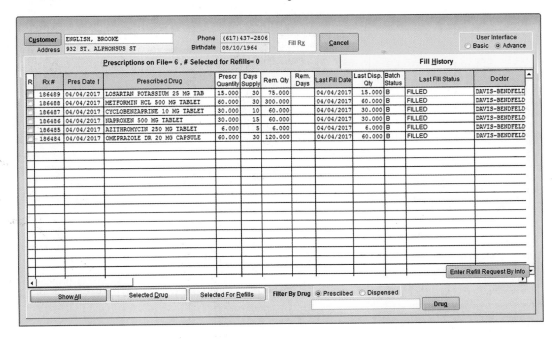

7. Using the form provided in Lab 50, complete a medication reconciliation form, and ask your partner to check this against your **PRNT SCRN** document.

8. Once it is completed, click **CANCEL** and close the *Prescription Processing* dialog box. You will be returned to the main screen of Visual SuperScript.

9. Click on the **Customers** icon on the left, and look up the patient history screen using the first three letters of the last name.

Enter *ENG* for English, Brooke.

10. Click on each tab at the bottom, starting with **Allergies**. Review this section by clicking on the various tabs. Record information for allergies, diseases, and diet, as well as for laboratory, miscellaneous, and any other required information to complete the form.

11. Together with the printed screen of the **Cus History/Refill** tab, include the completed medication reconciliation form for a final check by the pharmacist (instructor).

> ▷ **LAB TIP**
>
> Type in **CON** for *congestive heart failure not otherwise specified* and **HYP** for *hypertension not otherwise specified*.

EXERCISE

For the following patient: *Michael Duke, DOB 2.12.45*

1. Add the allergy to sulfonamide (SULFA) drugs to the profile.

2. Add the recent discharge information to the profile.

Add disease states *CHF, HBP*.

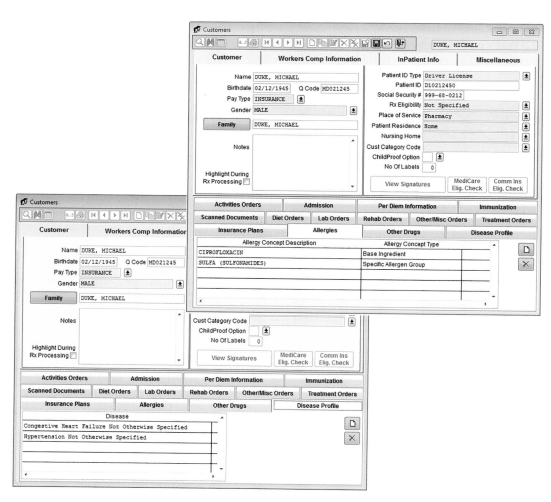

3. Verify with the patient (your fellow student) that all disease-related information is current in the profile. Use the **Prnt Scrn** function to share this with the patient for his or her review.

4. Complete the medication reconciliation report required for the institutional (hospital) record following the same instructions found in Lab 50. If you need pharmacology information, use a drug reference source.

5. Ask your student partner to review your completed form and your entry of the patient information before turning it in.

LAB 33

Entering New Intravenous Orders

▪ Lab Objectives

In this Lab, you will:

- Interpret a hospital intravenous (IV) order.
- Enter a new IV order from an institutional order.

▪ Pre Lab Information

Institutional pharmacy orders differ from prescriptions because the patient is considered *inpatient*, and any instructions related to patient care while he or she is staying in the health care facility are written on the order sheet. Other information such as laboratory work, diet, routine vital signs, and tests are included on the same order, and a technician must be able to pull out the medications. When entering a new IV order, additives and a base fluid will be listed. These components must be individually added and charged accordingly.

▪ Student Directions

Estimated completion time: 30 minutes

1. Read through the steps in the Lab before performing the Lab exercise.
2. After reading through the Lab, perform the required steps to enter compounded drug information.
3. Practice filling a prescription using the new compounded drug information.

STEPS TO ENTER A NEW INTRAVENOUS MEDICATION (DRUG)

1. Check your printer settings.
   a. Go to **OPTIONS** on the top toolbar of Visual SuperScript.
   b. Choose **RX LABEL OPTIONS**.
   c. Change *Label Type* to **TPN** (total parenteral nutrition).
   d. *WorkFlow Label* can remain as the default—**LM32**.
   e. Click **OK** at the bottom right of the window.

Rx Label Options

Label Type — LM32

WorkFlow Label — LM32

- ☑ PrePrinted Label
- ☐ Print Seperate Pat. Couseling
- ☑ Always Print Equiv. Drug Msg
- ☐ Print Lot #

Date Expiry Setting
- ⦿ Drug Days to Expire
- ◯ Lot Expiration Date
- ◯ Leave Blank

Customer Name Formatting
- ◯ Name As It Appears In Customer File
- ◯ First Name followed by Last Name

Label Setting for Pend Claims
- ◯ Do Not Print Any Label for Pending Claims
- ⦿ Print Regular Rx Label For Pending Claims
- ◯ Print Modified Rx Label Indicating "Pending Rx"

Equiv. Drug Message — EQUIV. TO
Rx Expire Message — USE BEFORE
Spanish Alt Lang # — 1

Label LM32 Settings
- ☐ Print Pat. Counseling for New Rx
- ☐ Print Pat. Counseling for Refill
- ☑ Print Pat. Counseling On Copies
- ☐ Print Pharmacy NABP #
- ☐ Print Prescriber DEA#
- ☑ Print Discount Message
- ☑ Print Days Supply
- ☐ Print Doctor Address
- ☐ Print Drug Description
- ☑ Print Rx On Hold
- ☐ Print Card Holder ID
- ☐ Print Price
- ☐ Print Price Captions
- ☐ Price U&C Price
- ☑ Print NDC
- ☐ Print Bar Code Rx No
- ☐ Print Bar Code Quantity
- ☑ Print Bar Code NDC
- ☐ Bar Code for Tablet Counting
- ☑ Print Warning Labels
- ☐ Print Gen. Name for Single Ingr.
- ☐ Print Physician Assistant Name
- ☐ Print Insurance Saved You Msg
- ☐ Print Date Of Birth On Receipt
- ☐ Print Patient Name on SigLog
- ☐ Print Remaining Qty

Promotion Message

[Save]   [Cancel]

---

2. Access the main screen of Visual SuperScript.

3. Click on the **DRUG** button on the left side of the screen. The *Drugs* dialog box will pop up.

4. Click the **NEW** ▢ icon located on the toolbar at the top of the *Drugs* dialog box. The form is now ready for you to enter information concerning the compounded drug.

5. Click on the *Label Name* data entry field. This text box will appear in blue when text is ready to be added.

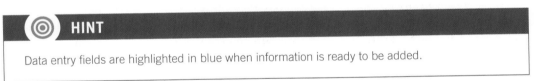

HINT

Data entry fields are highlighted in blue when information is ready to be added.

6. Type in the name of the compounded IV order that will appear on the IV label.

Enter D5WVAN50.

Note: *D5W* means *dextrose 5% with water*.

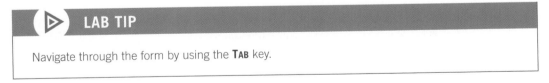

LAB TIP

Navigate through the form by using the **TAB** key.

7. Type your quick code into the *Quick Code* data entry field.

Enter D5VAN500.

Note: The *Quick Code* field is a useful tool to expedite the search for drugs in your database. The codes that you enter for your new compound should be based on the label name of the compound.

8. Click on the arrow to the right of *Drug Class* field. The *Drug Class* dialog box appears. Click on the appropriate drug class from the drop-down list. Click **OK**.

Select Rx.

9. Click on the arrow to the right of *Item Type*. A list of drug items appears.

Click on Compound from this list.

10. Indicate whether the new compound is gender-specific in the *Gender* field. Click on the arrow to the right of the *Gender* field to access the drop-down list.

Select both.

11. Tab to the *Brand/Generic* field. Click on the arrow to the right of the field. Identify the new compound as brand- or generic-specific by clicking on the appropriate choice.

Select Generic.

12. Click on the arrow to the right of the *Drug Unit* field. The *Dispensing Unit* dialog box appears. Click on the appropriate dispensing unit from the list. Click **OK**.

Select ML.

Note: *EA* means *each*; *GM* means *gram*; *ML* means *milliliter*.

13. Click on the arrow to the right of *Units*. The *Units* dialog box appears. Click on the appropriate unit from this list. Click **OK**.

Select ML.

14. Tab to the *Package Size* field.

Enter *250 mL* for package size.

15. Tab to *Days to Expire*.

Enter *14 days*.

 HINT

Vancomycin IV per manufacturer's recommendations has an expiration date of 14 days refrigerated and 7 days at room temperature. You may use a drug reference source to obtain this information.

MEDICATION SAFETY CONSIDERATION

IV large volume bags are hung for a maximum of 24 hours because of the breakdown of ingredients. The physician's order will supply the milliliters or milligrams per hour needed, and this rate will determine the time it will take for the IV to enter the body.

---

16. Click on the *Default Sig* field. This new compound may be frequently prescribed with the same instructions for use. Enter the appropriate instructions for use in the text field. If needed, these default instructions may be changed when filling the prescription.

Enter *Infuse at 125 mL/hr*.

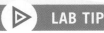
17. Click on the **SAVE** 💾 icon located at the top right of the toolbar. Basic information regarding the new compound has now been saved to the *Drugs* form.

18. You are now ready to add the *additive* ingredients of the new compound to the *Drugs* form. The bottom section of the *Drugs* form has three tabbed pages: (1) **MANUFACTURING & AVAILABLE NDCs**; (2) **COMPOUND DRUG INGREDIENTS**; and (3) **3RD PARTY NDC PREFERENCES**.

    Note: *NDC* means *National Drug Code.*

    Click the COMPOUND DRUG INGREDIENTS.

19. Each additive and amount needed in the new compound will be added one at a time to the grid. Click on the **NEW** 🗋 icon located at the bottom right of this *Drugs* form. Two dialog boxes pop up on the screen: *Drug Name Lookup* and *Compound Drug Ingredients.*

20. Type in the first few letters of the desired drug ingredient. Select the correct drug from the list by clicking on the drug name. Click **OK**.

    Enter *DEX* for dextrose 5% in water solution 250 mL (base fluid).

21. Enter the quantity needed for the dextrose 5% in water solution.

    Enter *250 mL*.

22. Click the **SAVE** button at the bottom of the *Compound Drug Ingredients* dialog box.

23. Continue to add each *additive* ingredient one at a time by clicking on the **NEW** 🗋 icon located at the bottom right of this *Drugs* form. Review the previous steps to add each ingredient. For this bag, there is only one additive.

    Enter *VAN* to perform a search for vancomycin 500 mg vial.

24. Enter the quantity needed for the magnesium sulfate, based on previous calculations.

    Enter *10 mL* and save.

Institutional Pharmacy Practice

25. Click on the **CLOSE** 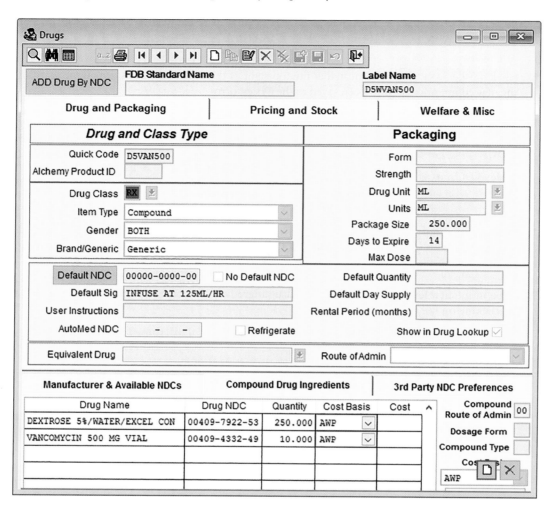 icon located at the top right of the toolbar. You have completed the task of adding a new IV order to the pharmacy computer system!

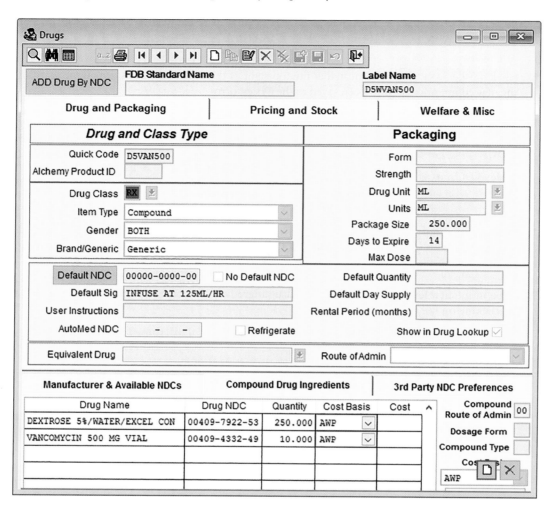

26. You are now returned to the main screen. Perform the drug look-up procedure to confirm that the new compound has been correctly added to the computer system.

   a. Click on the **DRUG** button on the left side of the screen.

   b. Click the **FIND** 🔍 icon located at the top left of the toolbar.

   c. The *Drug Name Lookup* dialog box appears. Type in the label name of the new compound.

        Enter *DEX* to search for Dextrose 5% with 500 mg vancomycin,
            or use the quick code you selected—*D5VAN500*.

   d. Select the correct compound from the list by clicking on the drug name. Click **OK**.

        Print the screen, and save it for your instructor.

   e. Read through the *Drugs* form to check for accuracy.

   f. Click on the **CLOSE** 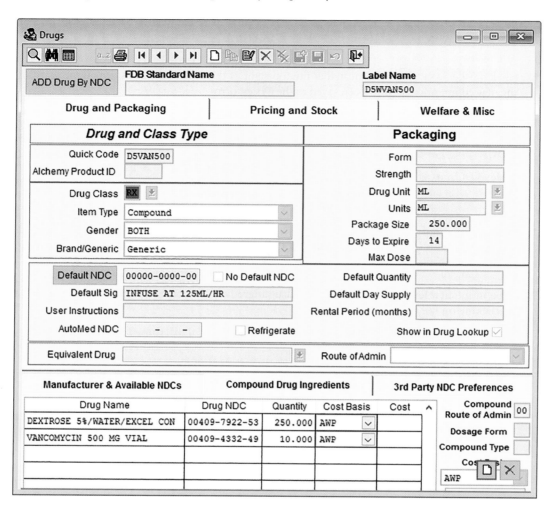 icon on the top right of the toolbar to clear the screen.

STEPS TO ENTER A NEW INTRAVENOUS
MEDICATION FOR A PATIENT
(CREATE A LABEL FOR THE IV ORDER)

Patient Name	Diet	Weight	Height	
Myrtle York	REG	134 lb	64	
Room Number	**Diagnosis**			
420				
Hospital Number	R/O sepsis, dehydration			
123334				
Attending Physician	**Drug Allergies**			
Stephen Hardy	NKDA			

DATE	TIME		
5/19	0615	*Admit to CCU*	
		D5W 250 mL w/vancomycin 500 mg IV q12h x 7 days	
		—— *v/o K Davis, RN. 5/19 0620*	

1. Using the steps in the prescription entry process (Lab 6), enter the IV order for the patient on the previous page.

2. When adding the prescribed drug, use the drug quick code created for the bag.

   Enter *D5VAN500.*

3. Once all information is added, print a label for the patient when all of the information is entered.

EXERCISES

1. Change the label type back to **TPN**. Using the following five physician orders, add each drug (IV medication) one at a time to the **DRUG** database using the previous directions for adding a new IV medication (drug).

2. You must choose the stock additive from the database and then calculate the milliliters needed to prepare the IV, based on the hospital orders (refer to previous steps).

 LAB TIP

Once the drug is entered, perform a drug look-up procedure to confirm that the new IV drug compound has been correctly added to the computer system. Once the drug has been entered, write down the quick code for each drug.

3. Ensure the label type is set to **LM32**, and fill the medication orders for the specific patients by following the instructions found in Lab 6 prescription processing.

MEDICATION SAFETY CONSIDERATION

Remember to use any approved reference for storage, dilution, and any special instructions needed for preparation. Once you have prepared a label using the steps in this Lab, prepare the IV order using the aseptic technique.

Institutional Pharmacy Practice

Patient Name	Diet	Weight	Height	
Ernest Hatcher	Cl liq	180	5'7"	BD: 3-27-29
Room Number	**Diagnosis**			
221-C				
Hospital Number	Diverticulitis			
47411 – Coolidge N.H.				
Attending Physician	**Drug Allergies**			
Dr. Terry Alexander	NKA			

DATE	TIME		
3/8/17	0715	NS 1 l @ 75 ml/hr	
		Zosyn 3.375 g IVPB q 6 hr	1st dose now
		Flagyl 500mg IVPB q 12 hrs	1st dose now
		CBC, BMP in Am	
		V/S q 4 hrs.	
		Tylenol g ÷ po q 4 hr PRN T ≥ 101	
		Dr. Terry Alexander, MD.	
		– 0710	

Patient Name Thelma Richey	Diet Reg	Weight 129 lbs.	Height 4"11	BD: 5-17-21
Room Number 321-B	Diagnosis			
Hospital Number Coolidge Nursing Home	Sepsis, R/o meningitis			
Attending Physician Dr. Mark Owens	Drug Allergies PCN, Sulfa			

DATE	TIME		
1/24/17	0730	Gentamycin 55mg / NS 50ml IVPB now	
		Percocet 5mg po q6h prn pain	
			V/o KDavis RN.
	1010	Admit to floor	
		Zantac 50mg / NS 50ml x1 Bag	
		Bicitra 15ml po x1	
		Reglan 10mg IVP now	
		CXR in AM - portable	
		BMP, CBC, peak & trough in Am	
		I / O q shift	
		Bedrest	
			V/o KDav RN

Patient Name		Diet	Weight	Height
Mark Ianella 9-11-63		Reg as tol	129	60 in.
Room Number 422-B		Diagnosis		
Hospital Number 74113		Failure to Thrive, dehydration		
Attending Physician Dr. Babu		Drug Allergies NKA		

DATE	TIME		
7/4/17	2200	Admit for observation	
		Condition: guarded.	
		Ensure upon admit.	
		NS 1 l @ 125 ml hr c̄ MVI	
		Kdur 1 po now	
		CMP, CBC in Am	
		chest CT SCAN now	
		Levaquin 500 mg IVPB now and	
		in Am	
		vital signs q shift	
		Demerol 25 mg q6 prn pain	
		Phenergan 12.5 mg q6 prn nausea	
		V/o Dr. Babu	
		KDen, RN	

Patient Name _Mary Harrison_	Diet _Reg_	Weight _171 lbs_	Height _5'5_	BD: 6/13/20
Room Number _CCU - 233_	Diagnosis			
Hospital Number _45456_	_Pneumonia_			
Attending Physician _Dr. Lane Alexander_	Drug Allergies _NKA_			

DATE	TIME		
3/3/17	1730	Admit to Floor	
		vitals q shift	
		Rocephin 500 mg / NS 50ml IV now	
		Xopenex neb q shift	
		Motrin 1 tsp. po tid	
		D5 1/4 NS c̄ MVI @ 60ml/hr	
		CBC in Am	
		Dr. L. Alex_____	

Patient Name	Diet	Weight	Height	
Gary Henderson	1600/no salt	490	60 in.	BD: 4-30-47
Room Number	**Diagnosis**			
228-A				
Hospital Number	CHF, obesity, DM type II, asthma by hx			
537118				
Attending Physician	**Drug Allergies**			
Dr. Fenstermaker	PCN			

DATE	TIME		
8/9/17	1750	admit to inpatient status	
		1) CBC, CMP, UA, thyroid panel	
		lipid profile, BNP on admit	
		2) EKG	
		3) Xopenex 0.83mg qid	
		4) Lasix 40mg IV on admission	
		Meds:	
		Colace 100mg ÷ cap BID prn constipation	
		Glucovance 5mg ÷ BID po	
		Lipitor 20mg ÷ tab qhs po	
		Flovent 110mcg ÷ puffs bid	
		Norvasc 5mg ÷ tab po qd	
		Coreg 25mg ÷ tab po BID	
		Dr. Walter Fenstermaker, MD.	
		-1756	

LAB 34

Entering Total Parenteral Nutrition Orders

■ Introduction

Pharmacy personnel prepare various intravenous (IV) admixtures that are based on the needs of individual patients who are unable to eat or receive adequate nutrition. ***Total parenteral nutrition (TPN)*** is a solution commonly made up of three base components: glucose, fats, and amino acids. Electrolytes, as well as other medications, will be added to the base TPN solution according to physician orders. TPN solutions can be up to 3000 mL and contain as many as 14 different components, based on the physician's order and laboratory work. TPN solutions are infused or administered to the patient through a vein. A patient may need a TPN for a variety of reasons—malnourishment because of illness, diseased state of the digestive system, or surgical procedures performed on the digestive system.

■ Lab Objectives

In this Lab, you will:

- Become familiar with the purpose of TPN.
- Learn how to add a new TPN to the pharmacy computer system.
- Learn how to calculate the amounts of the components and create a label for a TPN from a sample physician order.
- Work with another technician student to check each other's calculations and process labeling.

ASHP goals: 8, 12, 18, 22, 25, 28, 35, and 36.

■ Pre Lab Information

You have been provided a sample TPN to use to enter an order into the database and to prepare a label. Once you have learned those steps, you will use a sample order found in the Quick Challenge section. You must calculate each amount for the components and then prepare the label and bag for delivery.

■ Student Directions

Estimated completion time: 45 minutes

1. Read through the steps in the Lab before performing the Lab exercise.
2. Perform the required steps to enter the TPN information.

HT: **139.7** cm   WT: **51.8** kg   Patient: *Erma Campbell BD: 10/3/24*

Adult *Total* Parenteral Nutrition Order Form (Central Line Only)

Date 2/2 Time 0930	Is central line access in place? [ ] No [x] Yes Type **grosshong** Date placed **2/1/2017**

Please note: Prescribers must make selections in section 1-6 of form

1. Base Formula (Check one)	2. Infusion Schedule
[ ] Standard Base: dextrose 20% and amino acids (AA) 4.25% (D40W mL and AA 8.5% 500 mL)	Rate: **83 mL/hour**
[x] Individual base: Dextrose ___ % and AA ___ %: (final concentration)	**Cycling Schedule (home TPN only)** Cycle ___ mL fluid over ___ hours
OR	
Dextrose **70%** **400 mL** AA **10%** **500 mL**	Begin at ___

3. Standard Electrolytes/Additives	OR Specify Individualized Electrolytes/Additives		
Check here [ ]	Specify amount of electrolyte		Check all the apply
NaCl 40 mEq / L	NaCl **30**	**mEq / L**	[x] Adult MVI 5 mLs / day
NaAc 20 mEq / L	NaAc	mEq / L	[x] MTE – 5 5 mLs / day
KCl 20 mEq / L	NaPhos	mEq / L	[ ] Regular Human Insulin
Kphos 22 mEq / L	KCl **15**	mEq / L	___ units / Liter
CaGlu 4.7 mEq / L	KAc	mEq / L	[ ] Vitamin C 500 mg / day
MagSO4 8 mEq / L	Kphos	mEq / L	[ ] H 2 antagonist ___ mg / day
Adult MVI 10 mL / day	CaGlu	mEq / L	___ drug
MTE-5 3 mL / day	Mag SO4	mEq / L	[ ] Other additives
DO NOT USE IN RENAL DYSFUNCTION!	Maximum Phosphate (Na phos ___ 40 mEq / L or K phos 44 mEq / L ___ and maximum clearance 10 mEq / L		

4. Lipids (Check one)	5. Blood Glucose monitoring orders
Infuse lipids over 12 hours IV	Blood glucose monitoring every **12** hours with
[ ] 20% 250 mL every Tuesday/Thursday	sliding scale regular human insulin.
[ ] 20% 250 mL every day	Route (Circle one) **SQ** IV
[ ] 20% 250 mL every other day	**Sliding Scale** (Check one)
[x] Other schedule	[x] Sliding scale per T and T protocol
Liposyn 10% 100 mL	[ ] Individualized sliding scale (write below)

Additional Orders (All patients)	6. Routine Laboratory Orders (Check all that apply)
1. Consult Nutrition Support Team.	[ ] BMP, Mg, Phos every AM X 3 days then every Monday & Thursday
2. CMP, Mg, Phos, triglyceride, prealbumin in the AM.	[ ] Prealbumin every Monday
3. Weigh patient daily.	[ ] Metabolic study per RT (University only)
4. Strict I/O & document in chart.	[ ] 24 hour UUN and creatinine clearance
5. Keep TPN line inviolate.	
6. If TPN interrupted for any reason, hang D10W@ current TPN rate.	

Physician Signature *Karen Davis*

STEPS TO ENTER A TOTAL PARENTERAL NUTRITION ORDER

1. Check your printer settings.
   a. Go to **OPTIONS** on the top toolbar of Visual SuperScript.
   b. Choose **RX LABEL OPTIONS**.
   c. Change *Label Type* to **TPN**.
   d. *WorkFlow Label* can remain as the default—**LM32**.
   e. Click **OK** at the bottom right of the window.
2. Access the main screen of Visual SuperScript.

3. Click the **Drug** button on the left side of the screen. A *Drugs* dialog box will pop up.

4. Enter the TPN compound using the steps in Lab 33. Use the following steps to enter each ingredient for the TPN.

5. Type in the name of the compounded IV order that will appear on the IV label.

   Enter *TPN Base*.

6. Type your quick code into the *Quick Code* data entry field.

   Enter *TPN*.

7. Input the package size information into the *Package Size* field.

   Enter *1000* for 1000 mL.

   Note: This unit indicates a final container bag of 1000 mL or 1 L.

8. Click on the *Default Sig* field. TPNs may be frequently prescribed with the same infusion rate. If needed, these default instructions may be changed when filling the prescription.

   Enter *Infuse at 83 mL/hr*.

9. Click on the **Save** 🖫 icon located at the top right of the toolbar. Basic information regarding the new TPN base solution has now been saved to the *Drugs* form.

10. You are now ready to add the ingredients of the base TPN to the *Drugs* form. The bottom section of the *Drugs* form has three tabbed pages: (1) **Manufacturing & Available NDCs**; (2) **Compound Drug Ingredients**; and (3) **3rd Party NDC Preferences**.

    Note: *NDC* means *National Drug Code*.

    Select **Compound Drug Ingredients**.

11. Each ingredient in the new compound will be added one at a time to the grid. Click on the **New** 🗋 icon located at the bottom right of this *Drugs* form. Two dialog boxes pop up on the screen: *Drug Name Lookup* and *Compound Drug Ingredients*.

12. Type in the first few letters of the desired drug ingredient. Select the correct drug from the list by clicking on the drug name. Click **OK**.

    Enter *AMI for Aminosyn II 10% IV solution*.

13. The *Compound Drug Ingredients* dialog box remains on the screen. Tab to the *Quantity* field.

    Enter *500* for 500 mL.

    Note: This number indicates the amount of amino acid added to the base TPN solution: 500 mL.

14. Click the **Save** button at the bottom of the *Compound Drug Ingredients* dialog box.

15. Continue to add each ingredient in the base TPN solution, one at a time, by clicking on the **New** 🗋 icon located at the bottom right of this *Drugs* form. Review the previous steps to add each ingredient.

    Enter *DEX* for Dextrose 70% water IV solution 500 mL.
    Enter *400* for 400 mL.
    Enter *LIP* for Liposyn II IV fat emulsion 200 mL.
    Enter *100* for 100 mL.

16. Once all of the ingredients are added, you have completed the task of adding a base TPN solution to the pharmacy computer system! Click on the **Close** ![close icon] icon located at the top right of the toolbar.

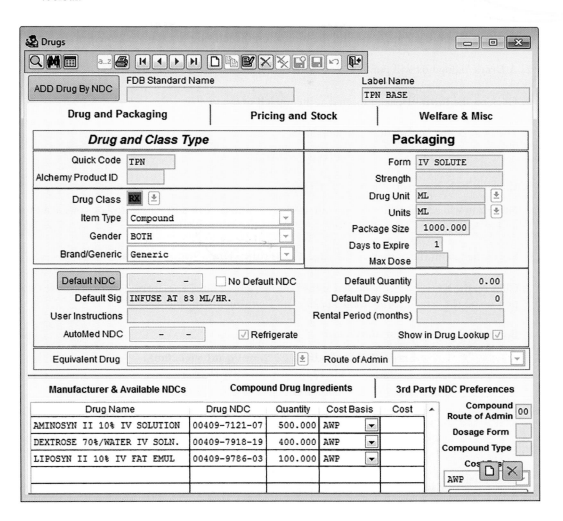

17. You are now returned to the main screen. Perform the drug look-up procedure to confirm that the new compound has been correctly added to the computer system.

a. Click on the **Drug** button on the left side of the screen.

b. Click the **Find** ![find icon] icon located at the top left of the toolbar.

c. The *Drug Name Lookup* dialog box appears. Type in the first three letters of the label name of the new compound.

Enter TPN.

d. Click on TPN base from the list. Click **OK**.

e. Read through the *Drugs* form to check for accuracy. Click the **Compound Drug Ingredients** tab at the bottom of the screen to verify ingredients.

f. Click on the **Close** ![close icon] icon on the top right of the toolbar to clear the screen.

STEPS TO ADD ELECTROLYTES

Add electrolytes to the TPN base solution, which will be determined by the order and the amounts previously calculated.

1. Click on the **DRUG** icon located on the toolbar on the left side of the main screen.

2. A *Drugs* dialog box will pop up.

3. Click on the **FIND** 🔍 icon located at the top left of the toolbar.

4. The *Drug Name Lookup* dialog box appears.

    Enter *TPN* for TPN base.

5. Click on TPN base from the list. Click **OK**.

    Note: You will see ingredients found in this base solution. Now add the electrolytes one at a time and in order.

6. Select the tab on the bottom of the page: **COMPOUND DRUG INGREDIENTS**.

7. Click on the **NEW** 🗅 icon located at the bottom right of this *Drugs* form. Two dialog boxes will pop up on the screen: *Drug Name Lookup* and *Compound Drug Ingredients*.

8. Enter the electrolytes into the record.

    Enter *SOD* for Sodium CL 2.5mEq/mL vial 20mL.
    Enter *12* for 12 mL for quantity to charge.
    Enter *POT* for Potassium CHL 2mEq/mL 10mL vial.
    Enter *7.5* for 7.5 mL for quantity to charge.
    Enter *TRA* for Trace elements add vial 5 mL.
    Enter *5* for 5 mL for quantity to charge.
    Enter *MUL* for Multihance 529 mg/mL vial 5 mL.
    Enter *5* for 5 mL for quantity to charge.
    Click the SAVE button at the bottom of this drop-down box.

◎ HINT

You must calculate the quantity to charge for each ingredient. This is done using the ratio and proportion formula.

For example, the quantity for the Sodium CL is calculated as follows:

$$\frac{2.5 \text{ mEq}}{\text{mL}} = \frac{30 \text{ mEq}}{x}$$
$$x = 12$$

The quantity for the Potassium CHL is calculated as follows:

$$\frac{2 \text{ mEq}}{\text{mL}} = \frac{15 \text{ mEq}}{x}$$
$$x = 7.5$$

▷ LAB TIP

If other electrolytes need to be added, then remember to add them one at a time by following the previous.

9. Once all of the ingredients are added and calculations are double checked, click the **Close** ![close icon] icon located at the top right of the toolbar. You have completed the task of editing computerized data to add electrolytes and other ingredients to the base TPN solution.

1. Fill the following medication orders. You will need to perform the drug look-up procedure to ensure that the new TPN has been correctly added to the computer system. If the new TPN has not been added correctly, then you will need to enter first the TPN as shown in this Lab. Then you can process the prescription for the individual patient and print a label.

2. Using one of the following three TPN orders, calculate the amount of grams and milliliters needed for the order, and complete and print a TPN label. Show your work.

HT: **133** cm   WT: **62** kg

Adult *Total* Parenteral Nutrition Order Form (Central Line Only)

Date **11-2-17**	Is central line access in place? [ ]No [✔]Yes
Time **0730**	Type **grosshong** Date placed _____

Please note: Prescribers must make selections in section 1-6 of form

1. Base Formula (Check one)	2. Infusion Schedule
[ ] Standard Base: dextrose 20% and amino acids (AA) 4.25% (D40W mL and AA 8.5% 500 mL)	Rate: **100** mL/hour_____
[ ] Individual base: Dextrose____ % and AA____ %: (final concentration)	Cycling Schedule (home TPN only)
	Cycle____ mL fluid over____ hours
OR	
Dextrose____ %____ mL	Begin at _____
AA____ %____ mL	

3. Standard Electrolytes/Additives	OR Specify Individualized Electrolytes/Additives	
Check here [ ]	Specify amount of electrolyte	Check all the apply
NaCl 40 mEq / L	NaCl____ mEq / L	[ ] Adult MVI 10 mL / day
NaAc 20 mEq / L	NaAc____ mEq / L	[ ] MTE – 5 3 mL / day
KCl 20 mEq / L	NaPhos____ mEq / L	[✔] Regular Human Insulin
Kphos 22 mEq / L	KCl____ mEq / L	**15** units / Liter
CaGlu 4.7 mEq / L	KAc____ mEq / L	[ ] Vitamin C 500 mg / day
MagSO4 8 mEq / L	Kphos____ mEq / L	[✔] H 2 antagonis **50** mg / day
Adult MVI 10 mL / day	CaGlu____ mEq / L	drug **Zantac**
MTE-5 3 mL / day	Mag SO4____ mEq / L	[ ] Other additives
DO NOT USE IN RENAL DYSFUNCTION!	Maximum Phosphate (Na phos) 40 mEq / L or K phos 44 mEq / L _____ and maximum clearance 10 mEq / L	

4. Lipids (Check one)	5. Blood Glucose monitoring orders
Infuse lipids over 12 hours IV	Blood glucose monitoring every **6** hours with
[ ] 20% 250 mL every Tuesday/Thursday	sliding scale regular human insulin.
[✔] 20% 250 mL every day	Route (Circle one) SQ (IV)
[ ] 20% 250 mL every other day	**Sliding Scale** (Check one)
[ ] Other schedule	[ ] Sliding scale per T and T protocol
	[ ] Individualized sliding scale (write below)

Additional Orders (All patients)	6. Routine Laboratory Orders (Check all that apply)
1. Consult Nutrition Support Team.	[ ] BMP, Mg, Phos every AM X 3 days then every Monday & Thursday
2. CMP, Mg, Phos, triglyceride, prealbumin in the AM.	[ ] Prealbumin every Monday
3. Weigh patient daily.	[ ] Metabolic study per RT (University only)
4. Strict I/O & document in chart.	[ ] 24 hour UUN and creatinine clearance
5. Keep TPN line inviolate.	
6. If TPN interrupted for any reason, hang D10W@ current TPN rate.	

Physician Signature

Institutional Pharmacy Practice

HT: **162** cm   WT: **49.5** kg

Adult *Total* Parenteral Nutrition Order Form (Central Line Only)

Date **7-7-17**	Is central line access in place? [ ]No [**✓**]Yes
Time **2213**	Type **Grosshong** Date placed **3-27-17**

Please note: Prescribers must make selections in section 1-6 of form

1. Base Formula (Check one)	2. Infusion Schedule
[ ] Standard Base: dextrose 20% and amino acids (AA) 4.25% (D40W mL and AA 8.5% 500 mL)	Rate: **83** mL/hour_____
[ ] Individual base: Dextrose **25** % and AA **5** %:	**Cycling Schedule** (home TPN only)
(final concentration)	Cycle_____ mL fluid over_____ hours
OR	
Dextrose____ %____ mL	Begin at _____
AA____ %____ mL	

3. Standard Electrolytes/Additives	OR Specify Individualized Electrolytes/Additives		
Check here [ ]	Specify amount of electrolyte		Check all the apply
NaCl 40 mEq / L	NaCl **30**	mEq / L	[**✓**] Adult MVI 10 mL / day
NaAc 20 mEq / L	NaAc **20**	mEq / L	[**✓**] MTE – 5 3 mL / day
KCl 20 mEq / L	NaPhos	mEq / L	[ ] Regular Human Insulin
Kphos 22 mEq / L	KCl **20**	mEq / L	_____ units / Liter
CaGlu 4.7 mEq / L	KAc	mEq / L	[ ] Vitamin C 500 mg / day
MagSO4 8 mEq / L	Kphos **20**	mEq / L	[**✓**] H 2 antagonis **50** mg / day
Adult MVI 10 mL / day	CaGlu	mEq / L	drug **Zantac**
MTE-5 3 mL / day	Mag SO4 **10**	mEq / L	[ ] Other additives
DO NOT USE IN RENAL DYSFUNCTION!	Maximum Phosphate (Na phos) _____		
	40 mEq / L or K phos 44 mEq / L		
	and maximum clearance 10 mEq / L		

4. Lipids (Check one)	5. Blood Glucose monitoring orders
Infuse lipids over 12 hours IV	Blood glucose monitoring every **48** hours with
[ ] 20% 250 mL every Tuesday/Thursday	sliding scale regular human insulin.
[**✓**] 20% 250 mL every day	Route (Circle one) **(SQ)** IV
[ ] 20% 250 mL every other day	**Sliding Scale** (Check one)
[ ] Other schedule	[**✓**] Sliding scale per T and T protocol
_____	[ ] Individualized sliding scale (write below)
_____	

Additional Orders (All patients)	6. Routine Laboratory Orders (Check all that apply)
1. Consult Nutrition Support Team.	[**✓**] BMP, Mg, Phos every AM X 3 days then every Monday & Thursday
2. CMP, Mg, Phos, triglyceride, prealbumin in the AM.	[ ] Prealbumin every Monday
3. Weigh patient daily.	[ ] Metabolic study per RT (University only)
4. Strict I/O & document in chart.	[**✓**] 24 hour UUN and creatinine clearance
5. Keep TPN line inviolate.	
6. If TPN interrupted for any reason, hang D10W @ current TPN rate.	

Physician Signature

HT: **152** cm   WT: **52** kg

Adult *Total* Parenteral Nutrition Order Form (Central Line Only)

| Date **3-3-17** | Is central line access in place? [ ]No [✓]Yes |
| Time **0645** | Type **Crosshong**   Date placed **3-2-17** |

Please note: Prescribers must make selections in section 1-6 of form

1. Base Formula (Check one)	2. Infusion Schedule
[✓] Standard Base: dextrose 20% and amino acids (AA) 4.25% (D40W mL and AA 8.5% 500 mL)	Rate: **100** mL/hour_____
[ ] Individual base: Dextrose____% and AA____%:	**Cycling Schedule (home TPN only)**
(final concentration)	Cycle____mL fluid over____hours
OR	Begin at _____
Dextrose____%____mL	
AA____%____mL	

3. Standard Electrolytes/Additives	OR Specify Individualized Electrolytes/Additives	
Check here [✓]	Specify amount of electrolyte	Check all the apply
NaCl 40 mEq / L	NaCl____mEq / L	[ ] Adult MVI 10 mL / day
NaAc 20 mEq / L	NaAc____mEq / L	[ ] MTE – 5 3 mL / day
KCl 20 mEq / L	NaPhos____mEq / L	[ ] Regular Human Insulin
Kphos 22 mEq / L	KCl____mEq / L	____ units / Liter
CaGlu 4.7 mEq / L	KAc____mEq / L	[ ] Vitamin C 500 mg / day
MagSO4 8 mEq / L	Kphos____mEq / L	[ ] H 2 antagonis____mg / day
Adult MVI 10 mL / day	CaGlu____mEq / L	drug____
MTE-5 3 mL / day	Mag SO4____mEq / L	[ ] Other additives
DO NOT USE IN RENAL DYSFUNCTION!	Maximum Phosphate (Na phos) _____	
	40 mEq / L or K phos 44 mEq / L _____	
	and maximum clearance 10 mEq / L	

4. Lipids (Check one)	5. Blood Glucose monitoring orders
Infuse lipids over 12 hours IV	Blood glucose monitoring every____hours with
[ ] 20% 250 mL every Tuesday/Thursday	sliding scale regular human insulin.
[✓] 20% 250 mL every day	Route (Circle one) SQ IV
[ ] 20% 250 mL every other day	**Sliding Scale** (Check one)
[ ] Other schedule	[ ] Sliding scale per T and T protocol
_____	[ ] Individualized sliding scale (write below)

Additional Orders (All patients)	6. Routine Laboratory Orders (Check all that apply)
1. Consult Nutrition Support Team.	[✓] BMP, Mg, Phos every AM X 3 days then every Monday & Thursday
2. CMP, Mg, Phos, triglyceride, prealbumin in the AM.	[ ] Prealbumin every Monday
3. Weigh patient daily.	[ ] Metabolic study per RT (University only)
4. Strict I/O & document in chart.	[✓] 24 hour UUN and creatinine clearance
5. Keep TPN line inviolate.	
6. If TPN interrupted for any reason, hang D10W@ current TPN rate.	

Physician Signature

QUICK CHALLENGE

Using the TPN order for Erma Campbell at the beginning of this lab, fill the TPN order. Make sure that the compound in the medication order has been properly added to the drug database. Print a label for the patient when all the information is added.

LAB 35

Entering New Chemotherapy Intravenous Orders

■ Introduction

Chemotherapy medications are often infused in a hospital, but they can also be given in an outpatient setting such as a clinic or physician's office. The physician's chemotherapy order differs from a prescription, because the dose is determined on the patient's weight in kilograms and is most often written as micrograms per kilogram (mcg/kg). If the patient's order is written during a hospital stay, then additional instructions related to the patient's care while he or she is staying is written on the same order sheet. Other information such as laboratory work, diet, routine vital signs, and tests are included on the same order, and a technician must be able to pull out the medications. When entering a new chemotherapy intravenous (IV) order, a chemotherapy drug (*additive*) will be added to an IV solution. These components must be individually added and charged accordingly. The following is an example of a chemotherapy order.

CHEMOTHERAPY ORDERS

Date of order 4-7-17	Time of order 1400	Day 1 of this order 4-7	Patient diagnosis Ovarian CA
Pt name Allen, Mattie	**Birth date** 12-20-31	**Cycle #**	☒ Central Line ☐ Peripheral Line
Actual Weight 46 kg	**Ideal Weight** 50 kg	**Adjusted Weight** 41.7 kg	**Height** 145 cm	**Body Surface Area** 1.45 m²

CHEMOTHERAPY ORDERS: For each drug ordered below, fill in all boxes on the corresponding line or indicate n/a if not applicable.

Chemotherapy Drug	Rec dose	BSA/kg	Dose to be given	ROUTE	RATE	FREQUENCY or day #	# OF DOSES
Paraplatin	AUC=6		450 mg	IV	over 30 min	Day # 1	1

PARAMETER(S)	Instructions (Check all that apply)	
	Call Case Mgr/Provider	**HOLD**
For absolute neutrophils count less than:	[ ]	[ ]
For platelets less than 100,000	[✓] RN Ellis, Mary	[ ]
For Mucositis Grade 3 or 4	[ ]	[ ]
For serum creatinine greater than:	[ ]	[ ]
Other:	[ ]	[ ]
Other:	[ ]	[ ]

Prescriber Signature (MD/PA-C/ARNP) Dr. Ronald Zimmerman	Attending MD Signature (*required prior to order submission*)
2ⁿᵈ Attending MD Signature (*required for non standard dose if documentation not available*)	Pharmacist Review Signature
Two RNs must verify dose of chemotherapy prior to administration of initial dose	Two RPhs must verify dose of chemotherapy prior to its dispensing initial dose
1.	1.
2.	2.

Date of order: **4-7-17**	Time of order: **1400**

PRE MEDS:

[ ] Dexamethasone ___ mg PO/IV 30 minutes before chemo   *usual range = 4-20 mg*
[ ] Acetaminophen 650 mg PO 30 minutes before chemo
[ ] Diphenhydramine ___mg PO/IV 20 minutes before chemo   *usual range = 12.5-50 mg*
[ ] Ranitidine 150 mg PO 30 minutes before chemo
[✓] Ranitidine 50 mg IV over 15-30 minutes before chemo
[ ] Other_____
[ ] Other_____

Emetogenicity	Minimal	[ ] No antiemetic premedication required
	Low	[ ] Prochlorperazine 10 mg PO X 1
		[✓] Lorazepam **1** mg PO X 1 *usual range 1-2 mg*
	Moderate	[ ] Ondansetron 16 mg PO DAILY 20-30 minutes pre-chemotherapy
		OR
		[ ] Ondansetron 8 mg IV DAILY 20-30 minutes pre-chemotherapy on Days 1 & 8
		PLUS
		[ ] Dexanethasone 20 mg PO/IV X 1 pre-chemotherapy on Days 1 & 8 *usual range 4-20 mg*
		[ ] Lorazepam _____mg PO/IV X 1 pre-chemotherapy *usual range 1-2 mg*
	High-Very High	[ ] Ondansetron 24 mg PO DAILY 20-30 minutes X 1 pre-chemotherapy
		OR
		[ ] Ondansetron 8 mg IV DAILY 20-30 minutes X 1 pre-chemotherapy
		PLUS
		[ ] Dexamethasone ____ mg PO/IV DAILY 20-30 minutes X 1 pre-chemotherapy *usual range 4-20 mg*
		[ ] Lorazepam 1 mg PO X 1 *usual range 1-2 mg*

AS NEEDED:

[ ] Prochlorperazine 10 mg PO/IV Q 4 hours PRN
[ ] Lorazepam 0.5-2 mg PO/IV Q 4 hours PRN
[ ] Diphenhydramine 25-50 mg PO/IV Q 4 hours PRN
[ ] Metoclopramide 10 mg PO/IV Q 6 hours PRN

OTHERS:

[ ] _____
[ ] _____
[ ] _____

[✓] **HYDRATION**   [ ] **HYDRATION NOT REQUIRED**

▪ Lab Objectives

In this Lab, you will:

- Interpret a hospital chemotherapy IV order.
- Enter a new chemotherapy IV medication (compound) from an institutional order.
- Prepare a chemotherapy medication aseptically for a specific patient using a simulated chemotherapy order.

▪ Scenario

You are working in a hospital oncology clinic today as the *chemo tech*, and an order has been presented for a new patient. You will enter the drug compound following the directions found in Lab 33. Following that, there will be some additional physician orders to enter and prepare using aseptic technique for hazardous preparations.

▪ Pre Lab Information

Review Lab 33 for entering a new drug (compound).

Estimated completion time: 30 minutes

1. Read through the steps in the Lab before performing the Lab exercise.
2. After reading through the entire Lab, perform the required steps to enter compounded drug information.
3. Practice filling a prescription using the new compounded drug information.

Physician Order

Room: 422

Patient Name: Ronald Gaston

DOB: 3/22/38

Prescribing physician's name: John Schoulties

Rx: Adriamycin 10 mg/NS 500 mL
Infuse over 60 minutes x 1 bag

No refills

STEPS TO ENTER A CHEMOTHERAPY INTRAVENOUS ORDER

1. Check your printer settings.
   a. Go to **OPTIONS** on the top toolbar of Visual SuperScript.
   b. Choose **RX LABEL OPTIONS**.
   c. Change *Label Type* to **TPN**.
   d. *WorkFlow Label* can remain as the default—**LM32**.
   e. Click **OK** at the bottom right of the window.

2. Access the main screen of Visual SuperScript.

3. Click the **DRUG** button on the left side of the screen. A dialog box entitled *Drugs* will pop up.

4. Enter the chemotherapy IV order using the steps in Lab 33. Use the following steps to enter each ingredient for the order.

5. Type in the name of the compounded IV order that will appear on the IV label.

   Enter *Adriamycin 10 mg/NS 500 mL.*

 LAB TIP

Navigate through the form by using the **TAB** key.

6. Type your quick code into the *Quick Code* data entry field.

Enter *ADRNS500.*

7. Input the package size information into the *Package Size* field.

Enter *500* for package size.

Note: This unit indicates a final container bag of 500 mL.

 HINT

For intravenous solutions, enter the *Days to Expire* as 1 day (24 hours).

8. Click on the *Default Sig* field. This new compound may be frequently prescribed with the same instructions for use. Enter the appropriate instructions for use in the text field. **If** needed, these default instructions may be changed when filling the prescription.

Enter *Infuse over 60 minutes.*

9. Click on the **SAVE** 🖫 icon located at the top right of the toolbar. Basic information regarding the medication has now been saved to the *Drugs* form.

10. You are now ready to add the ingredients of the new compound to the *Drugs* form.

Click to select **COMPOUND DRUG INGREDIENTS.**

11. The IV solution and the chemotherapy drug additive and amount needed will be added one at a time to the grid. Click on the **NEW** 🗋 icon located at the bottom right of this *Drugs* form. Two dialog boxes pop up on the screen: *Drug Name Lookup* and *Compound Drug Ingredients.*

12. Type in the first few letters of the desired diluents or IV solution being used. Select the correct drug from the list by clicking on the drug name. Click **OK**.

Enter *Sod* for sodium chloride 0.9% IV solution
and the quantity of *500 mL* (base fluid).

13. Now add the chemotherapy drug or additive by clicking on the **NEW** 🗋 icon located at the bottom right of this *Drugs* form.

Enter *ADR* for Adriamycin 2 mg/mL vial, package size 10 mL.
Calculate the amount of milliliters needed from the order provided.
In this case, the quantity is 5 mL.

14. Click on the **CLOSE** 🖫 icon located at the top right of the toolbar. Now you have completed the task of adding a new IV chemotherapy order to the pharmacy computer system!

15. You are now returned to the main screen. Perform the drug look-up procedure to confirm that the new compound has been correctly added to the computer system.

    a. Click on the **Drug** button on the left side of the screen.

    b. Click the **Find** 🔍 icon located at the top left of the toolbar.

    c. The *Drug Name Lookup* dialog box appears. Type in the label name of the new compound.

        Enter *ADR* to search for Adriamycin 10 mg/NS 500 mL, or use the quick code you selected, *ADRNS500.*

    d. Select the correct compound from the list by clicking on the drug name. Click **OK**.

    e. Read through the *Drugs* form to check for accuracy. Click the **Compound Drug Ingredients** tab at the bottom of the screen to verify ingredients.

    f. Click on the **Close** 🔁 icon on the top right of the toolbar to clear the screen.

16. Prepare and print the label based on the patient information on the medication order at the beginning of this Lab.

EXERCISE

Using the medications provided by your instructor, prepare the patient IV label and chemotherapy medication for the order at the beginning of the Lab, and obtain the instructor's check (simulated pharmacist review).

 LAB TIP

Remember to change the label type before printing the patient label for your chemotherapy once prepared.

LAB 36

Preparing Prefilled Syringes

■ Introduction

An institutional pharmacy often prepares certain medications ahead of time to provide ready doses of specific amounts. The 10-, 20-, or 30-mL stock vials of medications, such as normal saline (sodium chloride) or heparin are often *repackaged* in 3-, 5-, or 10-mL syringes and loaded in automated dispensing cabinets. This premeasured amount and/or milligrams of a medication provides a ready dose. Once a medication is removed from its original package, the expiration date no longer applies. Each repackaged medication is assigned a *beyond use date (BUD)*, based on guidelines set by the U.S. Food and Drug Administration (FDA) and the United States Pharmacopeia (USP) chapter 797.

■ Lab Objectives

In this Lab, you will:

- Enter new drug compounds for normal saline and heparin prefilled syringes.
- Prepare syringes from stock solutions (vials), and complete the required labeling and documentation.

■ Scenario

Today, you are working in a hospital in the dispensing area for the automated cabinet. The medical surgical unit nurse has called and stated that the cabinet is out of heparin and saline 5-mL syringes. Your task includes making a batch of five prefilled syringes of each medication for delivery.

■ Pre Lab Information

Using the provided stock vials of medications and supplies, prepare the syringes for delivery to the floor.

■ Student Directions

Estimated completion time: 30 minutes

1. Read through the steps in the Lab before performing the Lab exercise.
2. After reading through the Lab, perform the required steps to enter the compounded drug information.
3. Practice preparing prefilled syringes using the aseptic technique.

STEPS TO ENTER A NEW INTRAVENOUS PREFILLED SYRINGE

1. Check your printer settings.
   a. Go to **OPTIONS** on the top toolbar of Visual SuperScript.
   b. Choose **Rx LABEL OPTIONS**.
   c. Change *Label Type* to **TPN**.
   d. *WorkFlow Label* can remain as the default—**LM32**.
   e. Click **OK** at the bottom right of the window.

2. Access the main screen of Visual SuperScript.

3. Click the **DRUG** button on the left side of the screen. A dialog box entitled *Drugs* will pop up.

4. Enter the prefilled syringe order using the steps in Lab 33. Use the following steps to enter each ingredient for the order.

5. Type in the name of the compounded intravenous (IV) order that will appear on the IV label.

Enter *SOD* for sodium chloride 0.9% vial, package size 10 mL.

6. Type your quick code into the *Quick Code* data entry field.

LAB TIP

Remember to choose a quick code to help you find the compounded syringes once entered.

7. Input the package size information into the *Package Size* field..

Enter *5* for 5 mL (each syringe is 5 mL).

8. Tab to *Days to Expire*.

Enter the BUD assigned.

MEDICATION SAFETY CONSIDERATION

Always check the manufacturer information on storage and repackaging practices for a unit dose (repackaged medication). Assigning a BUD is regulated by the FDA; the specific instructions should be followed.

9. Click on the *Default Sig* field. This new compound may be frequently prescribed with the same instructions for use. Enter the appropriate instructions for use in the text field. If needed, these default instructions may be changed when filling the prescription.

Enter *Use as directed*.

LAB TIP

The administration will be specific for each patient once the syringe is removed by the nurse for a patient.

10. Click on the **SAVE** 🖫 icon located at the top right of the toolbar. Basic information regarding the new compound has now been saved to the *Drugs* form.

11. You are now ready to add the ***additive*** ingredients of the new compound to the *Drugs* form.

Click to select COMPOUND DRUG INGREDIENTS.

12. Each additive and amount needed in the new compound will be added one at a time to the grid. Click on the **NEW** 🗅 icon located at the bottom right of this *Drugs* form. Two dialog boxes pop up on the screen: *Drug Name Lookup* and *Compound Drug Ingredients*.

13. Type in the first few letters of the desired drug ingredient. Select the correct drug from the list by clicking on the drug name. Click **OK**.

Enter *SOD* for sodium chloride 0.9% vial, package size 10 mL.

14. Enter the quantity needed for *sodium chloride syringes, 5 mL each.*

Enter *30 mL.*

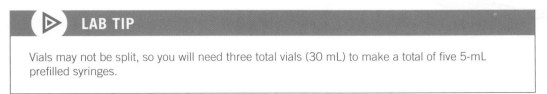

LAB TIP

Vials may not be split, so you will need three total vials (30 mL) to make a total of five 5-mL prefilled syringes.

15. Click the **SAVE** 💾 icon at the bottom of the *Compound Drug Ingredients* dialog box.

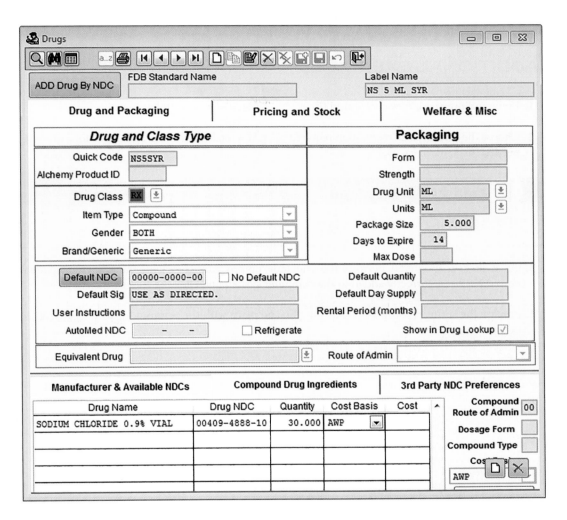

16. Click on the **CLOSE** 📲 icon located at the top right of the toolbar. You have now completed the task of adding a new IV order to the pharmacy computer system!

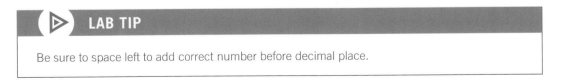

LAB TIP

Be sure to space left to add correct number before decimal place.

17. You are now returned to the main screen. Perform the drug look-up procedure to confirm that the new compound has been correctly added to the computer system.

   a. Click on the **DRUG** button on the left side of the screen.

   b. Click the **FIND** 🔍 icon located at the top left of the toolbar.

   c. The *Drug Name Lookup* dialog box appears. Type in the quick code you selected for of the new compound.

   d. Select the correct compound from the list by clicking on the drug name. Click **OK**.

   e. Read through the *Drugs* form to check for accuracy. Click the **COMPOUND DRUG INGREDI-ENTS** tab at the bottom of the screen to verify ingredients

   f. Click on the **CLOSE** 🚪 icon on the top right of the toolbar to clear the screen.

ADDITIONAL EXERCISES

1. Enter and prepare a new compound (drug) in syringes: Heparin, 100 units/mL.

2. Choose the correct stock medication required to make a total of five 5-mL syringes (a total of 25 mL needed for 5 mL in each).

 LAB TIP

Choose Heparin 100 unit/10 mL (10/mL).

3. Once the drug is entered, perform the drug look-up procedure to ensure the new IV drug compound has been correctly added to the computer system and click the **PRNT SCRN** key.

4. Prepare the syringes using aseptic technique, and place with the printout for your instructor to verify.

LAB 37

Validation of Aseptic Technique (Using Media Fill)

■ Introduction

When preparing intravenous (IV) bags for a patient, the preparer's technique requires testing or *validation* at certain intervals per the United States Pharmacopeia (USP) 797 guidelines. For low- and medium-risk IV bags, the validation interval is every year, and for high-risk IV bags, the interval is every 6 months. Employers must follow these guidelines when training, and the pharmacy technician student is often validated at the end of a course as well. Using kits that have a vial of a medium made of soybean extract is most common to test personal aseptic technique.

Before the actual preparation, the preparer must follow the required hand-washing and garbing (i.e., putting on the personal protective equipment [PPE]) processes. Once the bag is made, it is incubated for a period, following the kit manufacturer guidelines, to allow the bacteria to grow if introduced during the preparation process.

■ Lab Objectives

In this Lab, you will:

- Create a label for the IV bag before preparing.
- Complete a medium fill validation for personal aseptic technique.

■ Pre Lab Information

This exercise is your final validation of technique to test if bacteria are present in the prepared bag. You will combine all the steps learned from hand washing, garbing, and labeling, and use the medications provided by your instructor.

■ Student Directions

Estimated completion time: 15 minutes

1. Read through the steps in the Lab before performing the Lab exercise.
2. After preparing a label, perform the required steps for hand washing, garbing, cleaning the laminar airflow workbench (LAFW), also called the *hood*, and preparing the IV bag.

STEPS TO ENTER A NEW INTRAVENOUS MEDICATION (DRUG)

1. Check your printer settings.
    a. Go to **OPTIONS** on the top toolbar of Visual SuperScript.
    b. Choose **RX LABEL OPTIONS**.
    c. Change *Label Type* to **TPN**.
    d. *WorkFlow Label* can remain as the default—**LM32**.
    e. Click **OK** at the bottom right of the window.
2. Access the main screen of Visual SuperScript.

3. Click the **DRUG** button on the left side of the screen. A dialog box entitled *Drugs* will pop up.

4. Enter the compound IV order using the steps in Lab 33. Use the following steps to enter each ingredient for the order.

5. Type in the name of the compounded IV order that will appear on the IV label.

    Enter *PATT test* and your initials.

6. Type your quick code into the Quick Code data entry field.

7. Input the package size information into the *Package Size* field.

    Enter *100 mL* for package size.

8. Tab to *Days to Expire*.

    Enter *3 days*.

MEDICATION SAFETY CONSIDERATION

The PATT test bag will be incubated for a number of days to verify that no bacterial growth is present. Any bacterial growth would indicate that the preparer's technique when making the bag was compromised by touch or exposure to incorrect air.

---

9. Click on the **SAVE** icon located at the top right of the toolbar. Basic information regarding the new compound IV medication has now been saved to the *Drugs* form.

10. You are now ready to add the ingredients of the new compound to the *Drugs* form.

    Click to select COMPOUND DRUG INGREDIENTS.

11. Each additive and amount needed in the new compound will be added one at a time to the grid. Click on the **NEW** ☐ icon located at the bottom right of this *Drugs* form. Two dialog boxes will pop up on the screen: *Drug Name Lookup* and *Compound Drug Ingredients*.

12. Type in the first few letters of the desired drug ingredient. Select the correct drug from the list by clicking on the drug name. Click **OK**.

    Select PATT Media Fill Test.

13. Enter the quantity needed for the test.

    Enter *100* for 100 mL.

▷ LAB TIP

Be sure to space left to add the correct number before decimal place.

---

14. Click on the **SAVE** button on the bottom of the *Compound Drug Ingredients* dialog box.

15. Click on the **CLOSE** ▣ icon located at the top right of the toolbar. You have completed the task of adding a new compounded IV order to the pharmacy computer system!

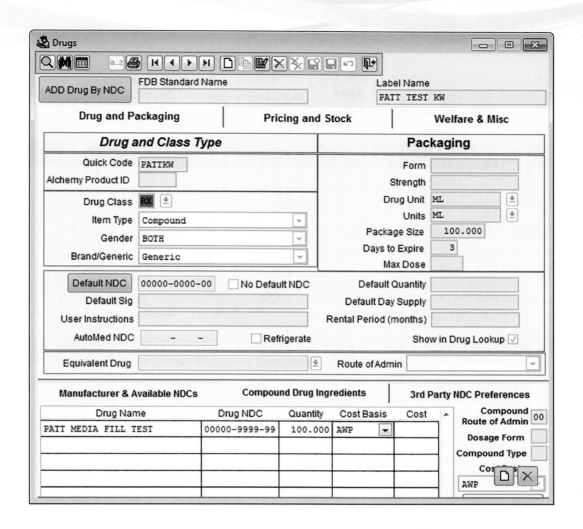

16. You are now returned to the main screen. Perform the drug look-up procedure to confirm that the new compound has been correctly added to the computer system.

   a. Click on the **Drug** button on the left side of the screen.

   b. Click the **Find** 🔍 icon located at the top left of the toolbar.

   c. The *Drug Name Lookup* dialog box appears. Type in the quick code you selected for the new compound.

   d. Select the correct compound from the list by clicking on the drug name. Click **OK**.

   e. Read through the *Drugs* form to check for accuracy. Click the **Compound Drug Ingredients** tab at the bottom of the screen to verify ingredients.

   f. Click on the **Close** 🚪 icon on the top right of the toolbar to clear the screen.

17. Print a label for the PATT test bag, and prepare the medication for delivery.

ADDITIONAL EXERCISES

1. Change the label type back to **TPN**. Using the following physician orders, add each IV medication to the *Drug* database one at a time to create an IV compound, following the directions for adding a new IV medication (drug) provided in this Lab.

 LAB TIP

Once the drug is entered, perform a drug look-up procedureto ensure that the new IV drug compound has been correctly added to the computer system. Once the drug has been entered, write down the
Q CODE for each drug.

2. You must choose the stock additive from the database and then calculate the milliliters needed to prepare the IV medication, based on the hospital orders (refer to "Steps to Perform a Drug Look-Up Procedure").

MEDICATION SAFETY CONSIDERATION

Remember: Use any approved reference for storage, dilution, and any special instructions needed for preparation. Once you have prepared a label using the steps in this Lab, prepare the IV order using the aseptic technique.

3. Change the label type to **LM32**, and fill the medication orders for the specific patients by following the instructions found in Lab 6 for prescription processing.

Patient Name	Diet		Weight	Height	
Ernest Hatcher	Cl liq		180	5'7"	BD: 3-27-29
Room Number	**Diagnosis**				
221-C					
Hospital Number	Diverticulitis				
47411 - Coolidge N.H.					
Attending Physician	**Drug Allergies**				
Dr. Terry Alexander	NKA				

DATE	TIME		
3/3/17	0715	NS 1 l @ 75 ml/hr	
		Zosyn 3.375 g IVPB q 6 hr ⟩ 1st dose now	
		CBC, BMP c̄ Am	
		V/S q 4 hrs.	
		Tylenol g i͞i po q4hr PRN T ≥ 101	
		Dr. Terry Alexander, MD.	
		— 0710	

Patient Name		Diet	Weight	Height	
Thelma Richey		Reg	129 lbs.	4"11	BD: 5-17-21
Room Number		Diagnosis			
321-B					
Hospital Number		Sepsis, R/o meningitis			
Coolidge Nursing Home					
Attending Physician		Drug Allergies			
Dr. Mark Owens		PCN, Sulfa			

DATE	TIME		
1/24/17	0730	Gentamycin 55mg / NS 50 ml IVPB now	
		Percocet 5mg po q6h prn pain	
			V/o K Davis RN.
	1010	Admit to floor	
		Zantac 50mg / NS 50 ml x1 Bag	
		Bicitra 15 ml po x1	
		Reglan 10 mg IVP now	
		CXR in AM - portable	
		BMP, CBC, peak ; trough in Am	
		I/O q shift	
		Bedrest	
			V/o K Davis RN

Patient Name		Diet	Weight	Height
Mark Ianella 9-11-63		Reg as tol	129	60 in.
Room Number 422-B		**Diagnosis**		
Hospital Number 74113		Failure to Thrive, dehydration		
Attending Physician Dr. Babu		**Drug Allergies** NKA		

DATE	TIME		
7/4/17	2200	Admit for observation	
		Condition: guarded.	
		Ensure aptn admit.	
		NS 1 l @ 125 ml hr c̄ MVI	
		Kdur ÷ po now	
		CMP, CBC in Am	
		chest CT SCAN now	
		Levaquin 500 mg IVPB now and	
		in Am	
		vital signs q shift	
		Demerol 25 mg q6 prn pain	
		Phenergan 12.5 mg q6 prn nausea	
		V/o Dr. Babu	
		KDer, RN	

Patient Name	Diet	Weight	Height	
Mary Harrison	Reg	171 lbs	5'5	BD: 6/13/20
Room Number	Diagnosis			
CCU - 233				
Hospital Number	Pneumonia			
45456				
Attending Physician	Drug Allergies			
Dr. Lary Alexander	NKA			

DATE	TIME		
3/3/17	1730	Admit to Floor	
		vitals q shift	
		Rocephin 500 mg / NS 50ml IV now	
		Xopenex neb q shift	
		Motrin 1 tsp. po tid	
		D5 1/4 NS c̄ MVI @ 60ml/hr	
		CBC in AM	
		Dr. L. Alex	

Patient Name		Diet	Weight	Height	
Gary Henderson		1600 / no salt	490	60 in.	BD: 4-30-47
Room Number		Diagnosis			
228-A					
Hospital Number		CHF, obesity, DM type II, asthma by hx			
537118					
Attending Physician		Drug Allergies			
Dr. Fenstermaker		PCN			

DATE	TIME		
8/9/17	1750	admit to inpatient status	
		1) CBC, CmP, UA, thyroid panel	
		lipid profile, BNP on admit	
		2) EKG	
		3) Xopenex 0.83mg qid	
		4) Lasix 40mg IV on admission	
		Meds:	
		Colace 100mg ÷ cap BID prn constipation	
		Glucovance 5mg ÷ BID po	
		Lipitor 20mg ÷ tab qhs po	
		Flovent 110mcg ÷ puffs bid	
		Norvasc 5mg ÷ tab po qd	
		Coreg 25mg ÷ tab po BID	
		Dr. Walter Fenstermaker, MD.	
		~1756	

LAB 38

Validation of Hazardous Preparation Technique (Using a Chemo Preparation Training Kit)

■ Introduction

When preparing *hazardous intravenous* or *chemotherapy intravenous* (IV) medications for a patient, the preparer's technique requires testing at certain intervals per the United States Pharmacopeia (USP) 797 guidelines. For hazardous preparations, the testing interval is every 6 months. Employers must follow these guidelines when training, and the pharmacy technician student is often validated at the end of a course as well. Using kits that have vials containing liquid that reacts to black light exposure is commonly used to test personal aseptic technique.

Before the actual preparation, the preparer must follow the required hand-washing and garbing (i.e., putting on the special hazardous protective equipment [PPE]) processes. Once the bag is made, the surface area, finished product, disposal of trash, packaging for delivery, and preparation technique are reviewed.

■ Lab Objectives

In this Lab, you will:

- Create a label for the IV bag before preparing.
- Complete a chemotherapy validation for hazardous personal aseptic technique.

■ Pre Lab Information

This exercise is your final validation of preparing a hazardous (chemotherapy) drug to test whether spray or spillage has occurred. You will combine all the steps learned from Lab 37, as well as hand washing, garbing, and labeling, and use the materials provided by your instructor.

■ Student Directions

Estimated completion time: 20 minutes

1. Read through the steps in the Lab before performing the Lab exercise.
2. After preparing a label, perform the required steps for hand washing, garbing, cleaning the biologic safety hood (BSC), and preparing the IV bag.

STEPS TO ENTER A NEW INTRAVENOUS MEDICATION (DRUG)

1. Check your printer settings.
   a. Go to **OPTIONS** on the top toolbar of Visual SuperScript.
   b. Choose **Rx LABEL OPTIONS**.
   c. Change *Label Type* to **TPN**.
   d. *WorkFlow Label* can remain as the default—**LM32**.
   e. Click **OK** at the bottom right of the window.

2. Access the main screen of Visual SuperScript.

3. Click the **DRUG** button on the left side of the screen. A dialog box entitled *Drugs* will pop up.

4. Enter the compound IV order using the steps in Lab 33. Use the following steps to enter each ingredient for the order.

5. Type in the name of the compounded IV order that will appear on the IV label.

Enter CHEM and your initials.

6. Type your quick code into the *Quick Code* data entry field..

7. Input the package size information into the *Package Size* field.

Enter 250 mL for package size.

8. Tab to *Days to Expire*.

Enter 1 day.

MEDICATION SAFETY CONSIDERATION

The chemo preparation kit uses vials of fluorescein dye that are only visible under a black light. The preparer must use proper techniques that eliminate any hazardous materials from being expelled into the air or on the work surface. This will ensure the safe handling and transport of the product.

---

9. Click on the **SAVE** 🖫 icon located at the top right of the toolbar. Basic information regarding the new compound has now been saved to the *Drugs* form.

11. You are now ready to add the ingredients of the new compound to the *Drugs* form.

Click to select COMPOUND DRUG INGREDIENTS.

12. Each additive and amount needed in the new compound will be added one at a time to the grid. Click on the **NEW** 📄 icon located at the bottom right of this *Drugs* form. Two dialog boxes will pop up on the screen: *Drug Name Lookup* and *Compound Drug Ingredients*.

13. Type in the first few letters of the desired drug ingredient. Select the correct drug from the list by clicking on the drug name. Click **OK**.

Enter CHE for chemotherapy kit 250 mL.

14. Enter the quantity needed for the test.

Enter 250 mL.

 LAB TIP

Be sure to space left to add the correct number before decimal place.

---

15. Click on the **SAVE** button on the bottom of the *Compound Drug Ingredients* dialog box.

16. Click on the **CLOSE** 🔣 icon located at the top right of the toolbar. You have completed the task of adding a new IV order to the pharmacy computer system!

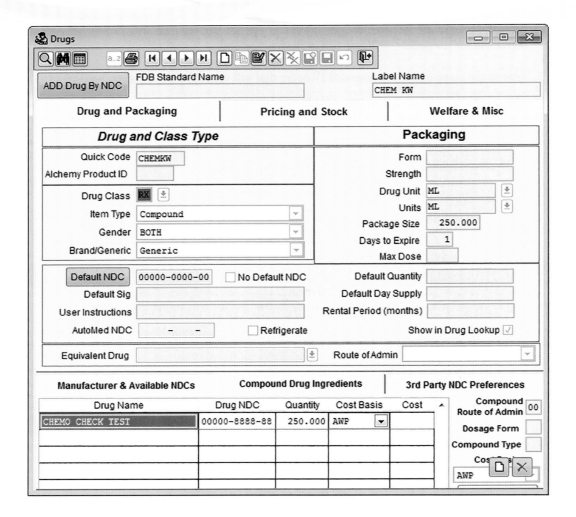

17. You are now returned to the main screen. Perform the drug look-up procedure to confirm that the new compound has been correctly added to the computer system.

   a. Click on the Drug **DRUG** on the left side of the screen.

   b. Click the **FIND** icon located at the top left of the toolbar.

   c. The *Drug Name Lookup* dialog box appears. Type in the quick code you selected for the new compound.

   d. Select the correct compound from the list by clicking on the drug name. Click **OK**.

   e. Read through the *Drugs* form to check for accuracy. Click the **COMPOUND DRUG INGREDI-ENTS** tab at the bottom of the screen to verify ingredients.

   f. Click on the **CLOSE** icon on the top right of the toolbar to clear the screen.

18. Print a label for the *CHEM* test bag, and prepare the medication for delivery.

Institutional Pharmacy Practice

Pulling the Pieces Together (Institutional Pharmacy Practice)

The Pharmacy Management Software manual is separated into pharmacy practice sections and is designed to teach the functions of automated simulation software by using detailed specific or isolated Lab exercises. Technicians in institutional practice work directly with patients, other inpatient departments or facilities, and physicians and nurses daily. Some of the tasks performed include:

Data entry and maintenance of electronic patient profiles

Emergency (disaster) preparedness

Medication reconciliation

Inventory control (automated compounding device [ACD], floor stock, emergency medications)

Reporting, returns, and recalls

Narcotic control and inventory

Sterile (intravenous [IV]) and hazardous compounding (total parenteral nutrition [TPN], chemotherapy, immunizations, and investigational

Medication preparation and distribution (repackaging, long-term care [LTC] blister cards)

Individually working through each task, starting with computer data entry and completing preparation of the medication with a prepared Lab exercise and list of suggested supplies (found in the Instructor Manual), allows skills to be practiced in a simulated institutional (hospital) laboratory setting.

Once the Lab exercises are completed, the program becomes the database label program to be used throughout the entire program for hospital and LTC exercises. In conjunction with the proper equipment and supplies, this program allows the trainee to complete and retain documentation of hospital and IV practice skills needed before entering the pharmacy workforce.

Institutional Pharmacy Practice

Institutional Pharmacy Practice (Comprehensive Exercises)

■ **Introduction**

The Pharmacy Management Software manual is separated into pharmacy practice sections and is designed to teach the functions of automated simulation software by using detailed specific or isolated Lab exercises. Technicians in institutional practice work directly with patients, other inpatient department or facilities, and physicians and nurses daily.

The Instructor should allow students to work through each task individually, starting with computer data entry and completing the preparation of the medication with a prepared Lab exercise and list of suggested supplies (found in the Instructor Manual) to allow each skill to be learned in isolation. Once these skills are performed, the Instructor should use the check sheet and associated documentation for each Lab as documentation for the student file.

The software manual provides times for each exercise, and should be used early in a pharmacy program for best results. Once the Labs are completed individually, the next step is to use the additional orders that can be interpreted and used in class activities in scenario form.

The form provided should be used to verify that the skills were learned in isolation and now are reinforced through practice in sequential learning. By using the software and skills learned, the daily activities common to the institutional setting can be performed in group activities in the simulated Lab. The program now becomes the database label program that is used throughout the entire program for hospital and long-term care exercises. In conjunction with the proper equipment and supplies, this program also allows the trainee to complete and retain documentation of hospital and intravenous (IV) practice skills needed before entering the pharmacy workforce.

■ **Lab Objectives**

In this Lab, you will:

- Use the skills learned to perform necessary computer functions to enter new IV orders into a pharmacy system.
- Use the knowledge gained to simulate real tasks, such as interpreting orders, using references for dilutions and storage, and using proper mixing techniques, performed in a hospital or institutional setting.

■ **Student Directions**

Use the orders on the following pages to simulate the processes of compounding sterile medications for hospital patients. You will interpret the physician's orders, input the data, and prepare labels for the IV medications ONLY. Use any approved reference to determine additional information needed. Once completed, your instructor may also ask you to prepare the IV medications using the aseptic technique previously learned in your program.

Patient name	Dennis Fulton	Diet As tolerated	Weight 201 lbs	Height 5'6"	BD 7/4/65
Room number	112				
Hospital number	332444	Diagnosis MVA			
Attending physician	Abbamont, Terrance				
		Drug Allergies NKA			

DATE	TIME		
10/31/17	1845	Admit to floor	
		ASA 81mg qd	
		Fe Sulfate 300mg sgr bid	
		Coumadin 5mg i qd	
		Diltiazem 120mg bid	
		Lanoxin 0.25mg i qd	
		Vicodan 5/500mg i q4 hrs prn pain	
		Ancef 1g IV q8 hrs x 3 days	
		Out of bed assistance prn	
		VS per floor	
		CBC and BMP in Am	
		CT left leg stat	

Patient name		Bernice Good	Diet		Weight	Height	BD
Room number		219-A	Reg		189lbs	5'5"	2/25/1918
Hospital number		332211	Diagnosis				
Attending physician		Alexander, Kelly	Pneumonia				
			Drug Allergies Estrogen drugs				

DATE	TIME		
12/28/17	0935	Transfer from nursing home via ambulance	
		CBC stat	
		Activity-bedrest	
		Atrovent 0.02% INH SOL per Resp tid	
		Colace 100mg prn q12h	
		Xopenex 1.25mg/3mL INH SOL per Resp tid	
		MOM 30mL prn q4h	
		Benadryl 25mg prn sleep	
		Nystatin susp 400,000 units S/S tid	
		Resp: 2L O2 via NC	
		Heplock	
		Dr. Kelly Alexander	

Patient name		Larry Jones	Diet		Weight	Height	BD
Room number		220-A	1800 cal ADA		130	6'0"	1/1/1929
Hospital number		322456	Diagnosis				
Attending physician		Alexander, Kelly	Osteomyelitis cellulitis				
			Drug Allergies				

DATE	TIME		
2/3/17	1830	Admit to floor	
		Up ad lib	
		Insulin Lantis 15 units hs (high alert)	
		Phenergan 12.5mg IV prn N/V	
		Morphine sulfate 5mg IV q4h prn severe pain	
		Vancomycin 1g/NS 250mL @125mL/hr q24h	
		LR 1000mL @75mL/hr cont	
		CBC, BMP in AM	
		Clindamycin 300mg/D5W 50mL @50mL q6h	
		If fever >102, Tylenol 1000mg po	
		—RBVO Dr. William Drake/ K Davis, RN	

Patient name		_Maria Rodriguez_	Diet	Weight	Height	
Room number		_321-B_	_3000 cal, reg_	_212_	_5'5"_	_7/12/56_
Hospital number		_233667_	Diagnosis			
Attending physician		_Alexander, Kelly_	_CVA, Alcohol abuse_			
			Drug Allergies _NKDA_			

DATE	TIME		
_3/30/17_	_0330_	_Admit to ER_	
		Begin banana bag 1000mL infuse over 2hr	
		Phenobarb inj 240mg stat	
		Dr. Alexander	
	_0610_	_Transfer to floor_	
		Assist with activity	
		D51/2NS with 20 KCL @100mL/hr	
		MVI qd	
		Phenergan 25mg prn q6h nausea	
		Tylenol 650mg prn HA/temp > 100	
		Maalox 30mL prn q4h GI complaints	
		MOM 30mL prn q6h prn constipation	
		Ativan 2mg prn IV or PO per scale	
		Phenobarb inj 240mg prn q3h prn convulsions	
		ASA 325mg qam	
		Plavix 75mg qd	
		Lovenox 40mg inj qd	
		Dr. Alexander	

Patient name		John Rogers	Diet		Weight	Height	BD
Room number		321-B	cardiac		212	6'1"	1/1/49
Hospital number		233667	Diagnosis				
Attending physician		Alexander, Kelly	CHF, HTN				
			Drug Allergies PCN				

DATE	TIME		
6/6/17	0330	Dx: HTN, CHF	
		Condition: stable	
		VS: qshift : continuous telemetry	
		Allergy: PCN	
		Resp:2L 02via NC, >94%	
		IV: 1L NS over 1h, then 75L/Hr	
		Lasix 40mg IV now	
		Cardiac enzymes q8 x2	
		CBC, UA this AM	
		Xanax 1mg po prn q6h	
		RBVO Dr. Unger/ K. Davis, RN	

Section III

Additional Practice Settings

INTRODUCTION TO THE WORKFLOW OF LONG-TERM CARE, MAIL ORDER, TELEPHARMACY, AND PRESCRIPTION BENEFITS MANAGERS

The Visual SuperScript manual is designed to teach the functions of several practice areas currently in the pharmacy practice. Technician training includes basic knowledge of the most common areas of practice, but, in addition to these, there are specialty areas.

Long-term care is becoming more prevalent as the population ages. Medications are packaged to ensure compliance and ease of administration. Strip packaging and 31-day blister cards are two common methods currently being used. Multitasking skills and critical thinking are key to these positions.

Mail order is another area into which technicians are expanding. Many organizations house their prescription interpretation in a separate area, such as the United States Department of Veterans Affairs (VA). Prescriptions are electronically processed and then sent to hubs for actual preparation. In addition, some companies and third-party insurance organizations process prescriptions for members by mailing them directly to the patient. Technicians must have good communication and reading skills and a solid knowledge of pharmacology for these positions.

Telepharmacy is a relatively new practice that some states allow. Terms such as *off-site support* and *remote-order entry* describe services provided by technicians under the supervision of a pharmacist who is not physically on site. This practice includes remote-data entry (often by technicians) and verification of processed prescriptions by a pharmacist. The combination of the shortage of pharmacists and rural areas provides a need for this type of pharmacy practice. Technicians must have good knowledge of pharmacology and the law, as well as good communication skills. The Lab exercises are designed to teach the skills needed to enter new prescriptions and to complete data entry functions.

Processing insurance claims, third-party processing, and working with prescription benefits managers (PBMs) are difficult and complicated parts of pharmacy practice. Some companies dedicate a whole arena or facility for just these tasks, and technicians are key to the industry. Working daily with health care professionals and correctly billing medications and services are the functions technicians usually perform. A solid understanding of terminology and pharmacology, good communication skills, and critical thinking are required in this specialty practice. The Visual SuperScript billing and inventory Lab exercises are designed to provide the skills needed for this area.

Using the database throughout the entire program in a simulated laboratory pharmacy, in conjunction with the proper equipment and supplies, allows the trainee to complete and retain the documentation of skills needed before entering the pharmacy workforce in all areas of practice.

LAB 39

Long-Term Care (30-Day Cards): Batch Filling for a Nursing Home

■ Introduction

In community practice settings, a separate business unit is often designed to provide medications for nursing or long-term care patients who are homebound. These orders are filled in 30-day cards or **blister packs** and delivered monthly or when requested, which allows each dose to be sealed into a separate cavity (blister). If changes occur, then the unused or unopened medications in the remainder of the card can be returned and repackaged based on the new order.

MEDICATION SAFETY CONSIDERATION

Providing a uniform way for medications to be packaged in individual blisters will ensure better patient compliance. The alternative is to provide a bottle of 30 loose tablets, which can be overwhelming for older adults or confused patients.

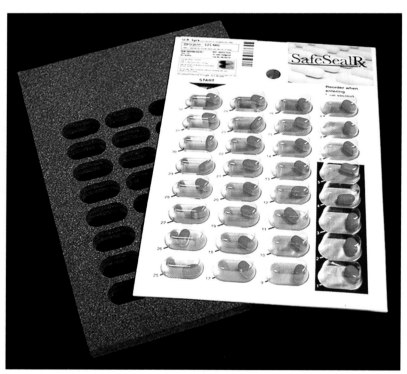

Courtesy Pearson Medical Technologies, LLC, Alexandria, LA.

■ Lab Objectives

In this Lab, you will:

- Learn how to process a group of prescriptions ordered for a nursing home, using a list and patient profile.
- Learn how to prepare the medications using blister packing.
- Learn how to prepare a report and medications for delivery or pick up for a nursing home.

■ Scenario

Mrs. Davis at the Coolidge Corner Nursing Home has called to ask for refills for some of the residents. She will send the driver around 4 PM to pick up the order.

Busch, Jane: losartan, 25 mg

Busch, John: lisinopril, 20 mg; pravastatin; 20 mg; and amlodipine, 5 mg

Fletcher, Irene: ofloxacin and atorvastatin, 20 mg

Richey, Thelma: lovastatin, 20 mg; loratadine, 10 mg; and alendornate, 70 mg

■ Pre Lab Information

Your pharmacy has a separate part of the business with contracts for nursing homes and long-term care facilities to prepare their residents' monthly medications. You will look up each profile and find the medications requested to prepare labels (refer to the same process in Lab 6). You will then put on gloves and pull the bulk medications using the National Drug Code (NDC) number verification process. If a person has morning and night medications, then they will be in different cards, one for AM and one for PM, similar to a daily pill box.

■ Student Directions

Estimated completion time: 1 hour

1. Read through the steps in the Lab before performing the Lab exercise.
2. After reading through the Lab, perform the required steps to complete the tasks in the scenario.
3. Answer the questions at the end of the Lab.

 LAB TIP

These blister pack cards may be **heat** sealed or **cold** packs, depending on the manufacturer. Either way, ask a fellow student to check your blisters before attaching the hard cardboard back and sealing.

TASK

You must first look up each patient and find his or her prescription numbers. Look for the most current prescriptions (dates). You will refill the prescriptions, prepare them using the blister packing method, and prepare a report for the resident's medications for billing.

Use the customer information on the previous page to complete the following steps for each customer.

1. Access the main screen of Visual SuperScript.

2. Click on **FILL RX'S** located on the left side of the menu screen. The *Prescription Processing* form appears.

3. Click on **CUS HISTORY/REFILL**.

4. Key the first customer name into the **CUSTOMER** data entry field. Press the **ENTER** key. The *Customer Lookup* dialog box appears. Click on the correct customer from the list in the *Customer Lookup* dialog box. Click **OK**.

Enter BUS for Busch, Jane.

5. Select the tab titled **PRESCRIPTIONS ON FILE**. Put a checkmark in the checkbox of the first prescription that needs to be refilled.

Check the box for losartan 25 mg.

6. Click on **FILL RX** located at the top of the dialog box.

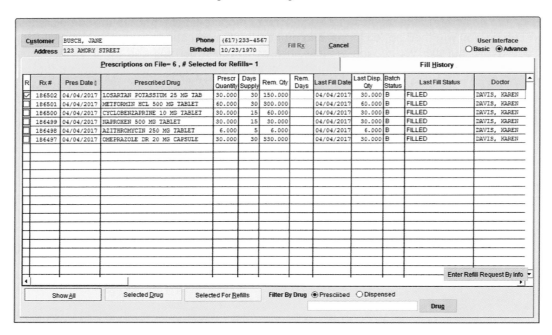

▷ LAB TIP

If the prescription has not expired and refills remain, then the *Prescription Processing* form is updated with the refill information. If the prescription has expired, then the *Cannot Refill, Select Copy Options* screen will appear. Complete the process of requesting refill authorization (see Lab 9) to refill each prescription.

7. The *Prescription Processing* form now returns to the screen. The medication checked in the box will be ready to process. Click on **Xmit/Record** located at the top left of the form, which will prompt the software to adjudication and print a label.

8. Continue with each patient's requested and specific medications by following the previous steps.

PREPARING THE REPORT

Once the medications are refilled according to the list provided by the nursing home, a report can be generated for billing and to verify each transaction.

STEPS TO PREPARE A BATCH REFILL REPORT

1. Access the main screen of Visual SuperScript.

2. Click on **Reports** from the menu toolbar located at the top of the screen.

3. Select **Customer Reports** from the drop-down menu. Then select **Customer History** from the expanded menu.

4. A dialog box appears. Note that the insertion point is in the first data entry field, *Date From*. Type in the date that the *Customer History Report* should start.

> **Type in the date when the batch was filled.**
> **The beginning and ending dates will be the same.**

 LAB TIP

Deleting the default date that appears in the data entry field is not necessary. The date that is keyed in will replace the existing default date.

5. The *Show* field will designate if the report should be generated to show the *copay* amount for the medications or the actual *price* of the medications. Click on the appropriate choice.

> **Select Copay.**

6. The *Format* field will designate if the report should be generated in an Insurance format or a NHome (nursing home) format.

> **Select NHome format since the patient is a resident of a nursing home.**

7. Select the *New Page for Each Customer* field if individual pages are desired.

8. The *For* data field offers several different choices in generating the *Customer History Report*. Select one of the five choices in which the *Customer History Report* will be generated. Click on the appropriate choice.

> **Select Individual Customer.**

9. The customer name entry field will ask for the customer name or the name of the insurance plan. The required information depends on the selection made in the previous step. Start with the first patient on the list:

> **Type in *BUS* for Busch, Jane.**

Customer History

Date From 05/16/2017 To 05/16/2017

Show ◉ Copay   ○ Price   ○ None

Format ○ Insurance ◉ NHome

☑ **New Page For each Customer**

For
◉ Individual Customer
○ Cust By Name Range
○ Cust By Insurance Plan
○ RX's By Insurance Plan
○ By Rx Statement Category
○ By Customer Category
○ By Customer State
○ BY Rx #

Customer Name BUSCH, JANE

Layout
◉ Portrait 👉
○ Landscape
○ Portrait Custom

☐ **Print Customer Address**
☐ **Print Authorization**
☐ **Print Disp. Days and Sig Directions**

To Send Email or Fax
Doctor Name [   ]

[Send Email] [Send Fax] [Preview] [Print] [Close]

[Generate Excel Format]

10. Click on **PREVIEW** located the bottom of the dialog box. The selected *Customer History Report* will open and appear on the screen.

11. Click on the **PRINT REPORT** 🖨 icon located at the top right of the *Report Designer* toolbar.

12. Click on the **CLOSE PREVIOUS** ⬐ icon located at the top right of the *Report Designer* toolbar. The report is closed out and the *Customer History* dialog box returns.

13. Follow these steps to create a report for each customer on your list.

LAB 40

Automated Strip Packaging: Batch Filling for a Nursing Home

▪ Introduction

In community practice settings, often a separate business unit is designed to manage the medication filling process for nursing or long-term care homebound patients. These batch medications are filled in strips with medications in individual pouches based on the times they are to be administered such as morning, lunch, and dinner, and delivered monthly or when requested.

For example, Mrs. Jones takes her Lasix 20 mg, Actos 15 mg, and folic acid 1 mg in the morning. All of these medications would be packaged in a single pouch, which allows the ease of opening one pouch for all of her morning medications.

Currently, the automated machines use bar code technology for verification by scanning the medications in bulk bottles and placing the contents in the canisters inside the machine. This allows each medication to be dispensed and then verified at the end of the process by the pharmacist's visualization and laser scanning of the packages themselves.

If broken or missing tablets are seen when the packages are being viewed by the laser, then the machine will stop and the pharmacist can pull the strip to correct the problem.

MEDICATION SAFETY CONSIDERATION

Providing a uniform way for medication to be packaged in individual pouches will ensure better patient compliance. The alternative is to provide a bottle of 30 loose tablets; for older adults or confused patients, this can be overwhelming.

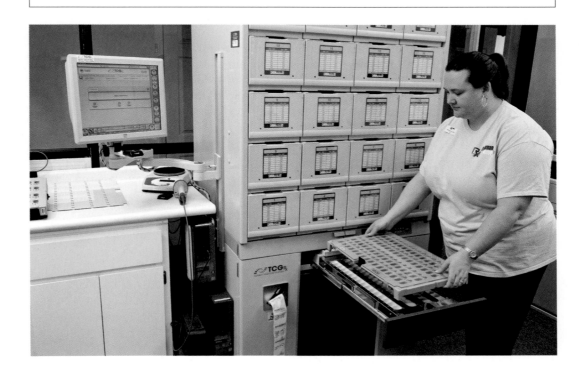

■ Lab Objectives

In this Lab, you will:

- Learn how to process a group of prescriptions that are ordered for a nursing home, using a list and patient profile.
- Learn how to prepare the medications using a strip packaging machine.
- Learn how to prepare a report and medications for delivery or pick up for a nursing home.

■ Scenario

Mrs. Nancy Davis at the Coolidge Corner Nursing Home needs the following monthly medications delivered to her home today:

    AM meds: Lipitor 20 mg; and Coumadin 1 mg

    Bedtime: Risperdal 1 mg; and Motrin 400 mg

    PM meds: Ferrous sulfate and hydrochlorothiazide (HCTZ)

■ Pre Lab Information

Your pharmacy has a separate part of the business with contracts for nursing homes and long-term care facilities to prepare their residents' monthly medications. You will look up the patient's profile and find the medications requested to prepare labels, which is the same process as Lab 16. You will then prepare the labels for each of the medications for a 30-day supply and package each medication in individual bags to simulate the packaging used in a strip packaging machine.

■ Student Directions

Estimated completion time: 1 hour

1. Read through the steps in the Lab before performing the Lab exercise.
2. After reading through the Lab, perform the required steps to complete the tasks in each scenario.
3. Answer the questions at the end of the Lab.

TASK

You must first look up the profile for the patient and find the prescription numbers. Look for the most current prescriptions (dates). You will refill the prescriptions and prepare them in three different single pouches or bags for morning, afternoon, and bedtime medications. Place the medications to be taken for each time in the respective bag. For example, if there are three medications to be taken every morning, place those tablets in the morning bag. Then prepare a report for the resident's medications for billing.

STEPS TO PREPARE LABELS FOR A BATCH REFILL

1. Access the main screen of Visual SuperScript.

2. Click on **FILL Rx's** located on the left side of the menu screen. The *Prescription Processing* form appears.

3. Click on **Cus History/Refill Rx's**.

4. Prepare labels for the batch refill referencing Lab 16.

LAB TIP

If the prescription has not expired and refills remain, then the *Prescription Processing* form is updated with the refill information. If the prescription has expired, then the *Cannot Refill, Select Copy Options* screen will appear. Complete the process of requesting refill authorization (Lab 9) to refill each prescription.

5. Each prescription chosen will appear in the Prescription Processing dialog box one at a time Perform the **XMIT/RECORD** process to charge to insurance and print labels to place on bags/ pouches.

6. Once the medications are refilled according to the list provided by the nursing home, prepare a batch refill report. Print for instructor validation. a report can be generated for billing and verifying each transaction.

Additional Practice Settings

LAB 41

Emergency Medications (Stocking an Emergency Box or Cart)

▪ Introduction

In the hospital setting, emergencies known as **CODES** often occur, during which a patient's life is suddenly in immediate danger. The medications required for a code are often kept in a special cart at the nurse's station. The pharmacy is responsible for the inventory of these carts. Once a cart has been used, it is sent to the pharmacy to be replenished or swapped with a fully stocked replacement. Each facility has a specific list of medications (**charge list**) that is kept in the cart. The technician will use this charge list to restock and check expiration dates each time the cart is used for a patient. Even if a medication is still in the cart, checking the expiration date will ensure that all items will be *in date* the next time the cart is needed. For any missing medication, the facility or the patient will be charged.

MEDICATION SAFETY CONSIDERATION

Because carts are not used every day, take out any medication that will expire *within 30 days* to ensure that the medication is in date when it is needed in the emergency.

In addition, outside health care providers rely on the pharmacy to supply medications. For example, the Emergency Medical Services (EMS) carries specific medications on the truck and must go to a pharmacy for replenishment after a call. The box is stocked with certain medications, depending on the area and requirements of the emergency service. A charge list of these medications is kept in the box, and a technician must replenish what was used and check for outdates when the cart is brought in. Once the cart or box is fully restocked, a breakaway lock will be placed on the container to ensure that the contents are available for the next emergency.

▪ Lab Objectives

In this Lab, you will:

- Demonstrate how to identify medications considered as *emergency* and the pharmacology associated with each one.
- Demonstrate the tasks associated with replenishing an emergency cart or box using a charge list.
- Demonstrate how to charge for the replenished items on the database.

▪ Scenario

You are working in a busy hospital pharmacy today and are responsible for restocking the emergency carts or EMS boxes. Using the knowledge and data skills you have performed to date, you will replenish each cart or box using the list provided in each and will use the database to charge for the medications used by filling the prescriptions for each medication.

▪ Pre Lab Information

Each technician should have basic knowledge of all common duties performed in a pharmacy. Regardless of the assignment area or practice setting for the pharmacy technician and pharmacist, everyone must work together as a team and help in an emergency. Although replenishing of code carts or boxes is a daily activity in an institutional pharmacy practice, it can also be sporadic as a result of emergencies. This activity will offer an opportunity to fill trays and boxes and to use the database for charging patients or facilities.

Estimated completion time: 30 minutes

Read through the steps in the Lab before performing the Lab exercise.
1. Using the charge list, check each item for its expiration date and current stock.
2. If an item is needed (because of expiration within 30 days or it is missing), then perform the required steps to create a label and to prepare the product for dispensing.
3. Once the cart or box has been checked by your instructor, place a breakaway lock on the outside and a blank (new) charge list inside.

STEPS TO ENTER MEDICATIONS USED TO REPLENISH AN EMERGENCY BOX FOR AN OUTSIDE EMERGENCY MEDICAL SERVICE

Use the annotated version of the Adult Emergency Box List below, along with patient information, that your instructor will provide. The list below is provided as an example of common drugs found in an adult emergency box.

Adult Emergency Box List

MEDICATION	VOLUME OF MEDICATION	QUANTITY	AMOUNT ON HAND	LOT NUMBER	EXPIRATION DATE
Infant 25% Dextrose INJ (250 mg/mL)	10 mL	2			
Sodium Bicarbonate INJ 8.4% (84 mg/mL)	50 mL	1			
Epi-Pen		1			
Atropine INJ (0.1 mg/mL)	10 mL	1			
Calcium Chloride INJ 10% (400 mL/mL)	10 mL	1			
Epinephrine INJ (0.1 mg/mL)	10 mL	1			
Dextrose INJ 50% (0.5 g/mL)	50 mL	1			
Fluids Available					
0.9% NaCl	250 mL	1			
5% Dextrose	500 mL	1			
0.9% NaCl	100 mL	1			
5% Dextrose	100 mL	1			
Supplies Available					
3-mL syringe with needle		3			
Alcohol swabs		10			
Huber needle and wing with on/off clamp		1			
Primary IV set		2			
Secondary IV set		2			

Filled by: _____ Checked by: _____ Date: _____

Additional Practice Settings

1. Access the main screen of Visual SuperScript.

2. Click on **FILL RX'S** located on the left side of the menu screen. The *Prescription Processing* form will appear.

 LAB TIP

> FIRST, check the stock in the box against the items on the list, and mark all missing items. EACH drug is then processed as a prescription (charged for) and added to the box. Remember to check ALL drugs and items on the list for the expiration date as well, and replace any drug or item that has an expiration date within 30 days.

3. Once you have identified the missing items from the emergency box list provided, fill a prescription for each item needed to replenish the emergency tray/cart using the specific prescription processing steps in Lab 6.

 LAB TIP

> In this case, the EMS service (customer) will be charged for the items used, and the patient will be billed from the EMS facility.

4. After completing the prescription processing steps, click on **XMIT/RECORD** on the left of the screen to complete adjudication and **LABEL/PRINT**.

 LAB TIP

> Printing a label for the medications needed will charge the facility for each medication used.

5. Place the medication in the box, and complete the charge sheet information. Affix a label to the back of the original charge sheet used to fill the box.

6. Repeat the previous steps to charge for other items that are needed to replenish the emergency box's stock.

STEPS TO ENTER MEDICATIONS USED TO REPLENISH AN EMERGENCY SUPPLY LIST IN THE HOSPITAL

Use the annotated version of the Adult Emergency Drug Supply List below, along with patient information, that your instructor will provide. The list below is provided as an example of common drugs found on an emergency supply list in a hospital.

Adult Emergency Drug Supply List

MEDICATION	VOLUME OF MEDICATION	QUANTITY	AMOUNT ON HAND	LOT NUMBER	EXPIRATION DATE
Dextrose INJ 50% (0.5 g/mL)	50 mL	2			
Sodium Bicarbonate INJ 8.4% (84 mg/mL)	50 mL	2			
Lidocaine 2% INJ (100 mg/5 mL)	5 mL	2			
Furosemide 20 mg (10 mg/mL)		2			

Continued.

Adult Emergency Drug Supply List—Cont'd

MEDICATION	VOLUME OF MEDICATION	QUANTITY	AMOUNT ON HAND	LOT NUMBER	EXPIRATION DATE
Atropine INJ (0.1 mg/mL)	10 mL	2			
Calcium Chloride INJ 10% (400 mL/mL)	10 mL	2			
Epinephrine INJ (0.1 mg/mL)	10 mL	2			
Vasopressin 10 mL	10 mL	2			
Amiodarone 50 mg/mL	3 mL	2			
Lidocaine HCL vial	20 mL	2			
Epi-Pen Trainer		2			
Adenocard 6 mg/2 mL (3 mg/mL)	2 mL	1			
Adenocard 12 mg/4 mL (3 mg/mL)	4 mL	1			
Nitroglycerin Sublingual Tablets (0.4 mg)	25 tabs	1			
Nitroglycerin Spray (Simulated 400 mcg/spray)		1			
Metoprolol	5 mL	2			
Solu-Medrol (125 mg/2 mL)	2 mL	2			
Aspirin (ASA) 81 mg (81 mg)	100	1			

Fluids

MEDICATION	VOLUME OF MEDICATION	QUANTITY	AMOUNT ON HAND	LOT NUMBER	EXPIRATION DATE
0.9% NaCl IV Fluid (250 mL)	250 mL	1			
5% Dextrose IV Fluid (50 mL)	50 mL	1			
0.9% NaCl IV Fluid (100 mL)	100 mL	1			
5% Dextrose IV Fluid (250 mL)	250 mL	1			
Nitroglycerin Drip (250 mL)	250 mL	1			

Supplies

MEDICATION	VOLUME OF MEDICATION	QUANTITY	AMOUNT ON HAND	LOT NUMBER	EXPIRATION DATE
3 mL Syringe 22 g x 1" Luer Lock		3			
5 mL Syringe 22 g x 1.5"		2			
Exel 10 mL Luer Lock Syringe 22 g x 1"		2			
MONOJECT SoftPack 35 mL Syringe		2			
Alcohol Prep Pads Medium 2 Ply		1 pkg			
B. Braun Secondary IV Administration Set 40"		1			
Medication Added Labels		1 pkg			

Filled by: _____ Checked by: _____ Date: _____

1. Access the main screen of Visual SuperScript.

2. Click on **FILL RX'S** located on the left side of the menu screen. The *Prescription Processing* form appears.

3. Once you have identified missing items from the emergency drug list provided, fill a prescription for each item needed to replenish the hospital's emergency supply using the specific prescription processing steps in Lab 6.

 LAB TIP

In this case, the patient is in the hospital and will be charged for the items used.

4. After completing the prescription processing steps, click on **XMIT/RECORD** on the left of the screen to complete adjudication and **LABEL/PRINT**.

5. Place the medication in the box, and complete the charge sheet information. Affix a label to the back of the original charge drawer used to fill the cart or tray.

6. Repeat the previous steps to charge for other items that are needed to replenish the cart or tray's stock.

Pulling the Pieces Together
(Additional Pharmacy Practice Settings)

The Pharmacy Management Software manual is separated into pharmacy practice sections and is designed to teach the functions of automated simulation software by using detailed specific or isolated Lab exercises. Technicians in additional practice settings work directly with patients, other inpatient and outpatient department or facilities, and multiple health care providers. Some common areas of practice include

Call centers (data entry, customer calls, and maintenance of electronic patient profiles)
Medication reconciliation
Inventory control (robots, automated compounding device [ACD], floor stock, emergency medications)
Narcotic technician (delivery, record keeping, inventory)
Sterile (intravenous [IV]) and compounding (total parenteral nutrition [TPN], immunization, investigational)
Sterile (IV) compounding hazardous medications (chemotherapy)
Nuclear pharmacy
Medication preparation and distribution centers (repackaging, long-term care [LTC] cabinets, blister cards)
Medication preparation and distribution (repackaging, long-term care [LTC] blister cards)

Working through each task individually, starting with computer data entry and completing preparation of the medication with a prepared Lab exercise and list of suggested supplies (found in the Instructor manual), allows skills to be practiced in additional simulated pharmacy practice settings.

Once the Lab exercises are completed, the program becomes the database label program to be used throughout the entire program for hospital and LTC exercises. In conjunction with the proper equipment and supplies, this program allows the trainee to complete and retain documentation of hospital and IV practice skills needed before entering the pharmacy workforce.

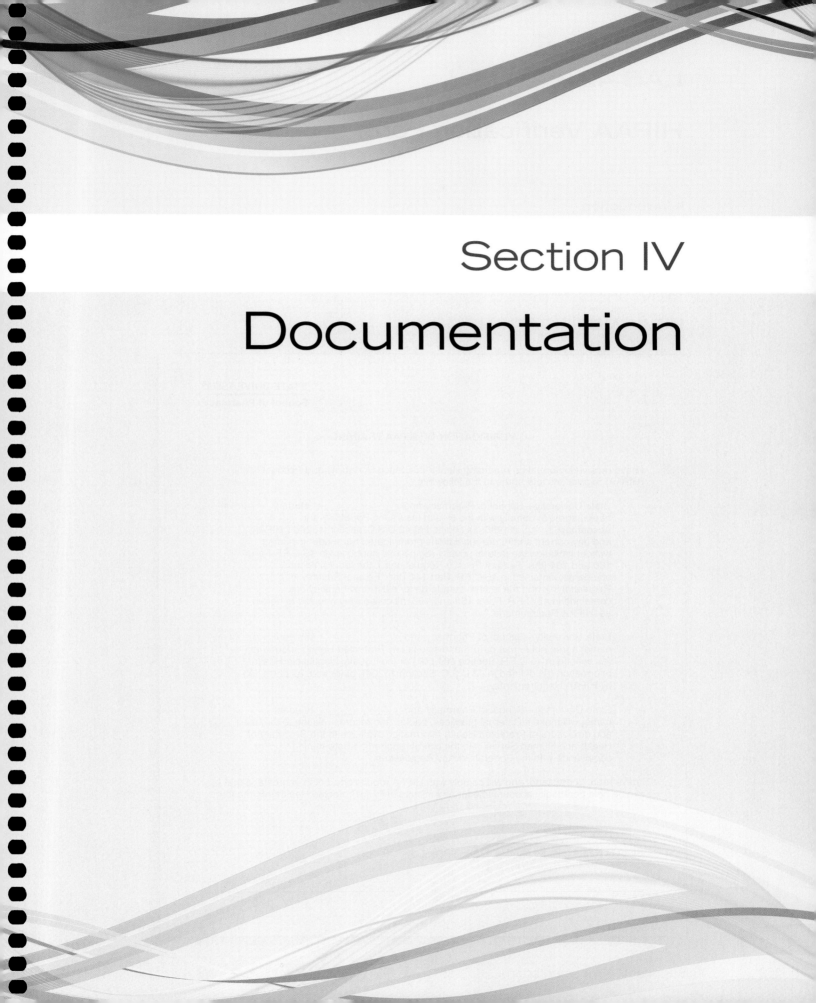

Section IV

Documentation

LAB 42

HIPAA Verification Form

■ Introduction

The Health Insurance Portability and Accountability Act of 1996 (HIPAA) was established by the federal government to protect patients' rights and the privacy of their health data. Most organizations require their workforce to complete HIPAA training. The form included in this Lab is an example of a form that staff members must sign to confirm that they received and understood their training. A copy of the form is available on the Evolve Resources site.

HIPAA VERIFICATION FORM

STATE UNIVERSITY
School of Pharmacy

VERIFICATION OF HIPAA TRAINING

I have received information regarding Health Insurance Portability and Accountability (HIPAA) regulations and agree to the following:

State University—School of Pharmacy and _____ [student name] agree to comply with the Health Insurance Portability and Accountability Act of 1996, as codified at 42 U.S.C. section 1320d ("HIPAA") and any current and future regulations promulgated hereunder including without limitation the federal privacy regulations contained in 45 C.F.F. Parts 160 and 164 (the "Federal Privacy Regulations"), the federal security standards contained in 45 C.F.R. Part 142 (the "Federal Security Regulations"), and the federal standards for electronic transactions contained in 45 C.F.R. Parts 160 and 162, all collectively referred to herein as "HIPAA Requirements."

State University—School of Pharmacy and _____ [student name] agree not to use or further disclose any Protected Health Information (as defined in 45 C.F.R. Section 164.501) or Individually Identifiable Health Information (as defined in 42 U.S.C. Section 1320d), other than as permitted by HIPAA Requirements.

State University—School of Pharmacy and _____ [student name] will make its internal practices, books, and records relating to the use and disclosure of Protected Health Information available to the Secretary of Health and Human Services to the extent required for determining compliance with the Federal Privacy Regulations.

I have read, understand, and will comply with HIPAA regulations. I also understand that I can be held personally accountable for any misuse of PHI (Protected Health Information).

_____
Student Name (please print)

_____   _____

Documentation

LAB 43

Prior Authorization

■ Introduction

A medication that is not one of an insurance company's approved medications may need additional documentation as to why it is being prescribed instead of an approved drug. A prior authorization form is needed to receive approval of the medication by the insurance company for a patient. Steps on how to process a new prescription for a prior-approved drug can be found in Lab 10, and a printable version of the form is available on the Evolve Resources site.

PRIOR AUTHORIZATION FORM

Pharmacy Prior Authorization Request Form			
Patient Information		**Provider Information**	
Patient Name:		Provider Name:	
Insurance ID #:		NPI#:	
DOB:		Office Phone:	
Phone:		Office Fax:	
Street Address:		Office Street Address:	
City, State, Zip Code:		City, State, Zip Code:	
Medical Information			
Medication:	Strength:	Route of Administration:	Frequency:
Is This Medication a New Start? ☐ Yes ☐ No		Directions for Use	
Clinical Information			
Diagnosis:	ICD-9/10 Code(s):	Height/Weight:	Allergies:
What medication(s) has the patient tried but with adverse outcome?			
Are there any supporting labs or test results? (Please specify)			
Are any other comments, diagnoses, symptoms, or any additional information the physician feels is important to this review?			
Provider's Signature:			Date:

LAB 44

Inventory Documentation

■ Introduction

Keeping track of a pharmacy's inventory is essential as items come in and out. The shipments pharmacies receive can be large and expensive. A sample packing slip list from a shipment is included in this Lab and on the Evolve Resources site.

SAMPLE PACKING SLIP LIST

MAIN STREET DRUG CO.
600 PHARMACY AVE.
NORMAL, GA 31600
PHONE: 800-555-6745

DEA #: RS0001234

INVOICE
Date: 12/6/16

PAGE	1
INVOICE #	6526769
ROUTE	3700
CUSTOMER	5555
INVOICE DUE DATE	12/20/16
TOTAL AMOUNT	2996.45

SHIP TO:
NORMAL PHARMACY
240 SECOND ST.
NORMAL, GA 31600

BILL TO:
NORMAL PHARMACY
240 SECOND ST.
NORMAL, GA 31600

CUSTOMER PURCHASE ORDER #				CONFIRMATION #		DEA 222 FORM #		CUSTOMER'S DEA #		ORDER #		
LTC9				5344				FD1234567		6886242-000		

CD	QTY ORD	QTY SHIP	PACK SIZE	U/M	DESCRIPTION	ITEM	NDC/UPC	RX	AWP	PRICE	AMT	COMMENT
	1	1	1X1000 TAB	EA	ALLOPURINOL TAB 300 MG OR/RND	082479	00603211632	RX	833.12	248.68	248.68	Contract
	1	1	1X12 CAP	EA	AMITIZA GELCAPS 8MCG	392506	64764008060	RX	396.32	330.27	330.27	
	1	1	1X15 ML SOL	EA	ARTIFICIAL TEAR OP SOL 15CC REPLACES ITEM 118208 NEW NDC	746404	30536108494	OT	4.38	1.35	1.35	Contract
	1	1	1X1000 TAB	EA	BENZTROPINE TAB 0.5MG	131342	00603243332	RX	386.25	93.05	93.05	Contract
	4	4	1 EA	EA	BUBBLE PAPER MAILER 7.25X11.25	585224	05113194534	OT	.00	.39	1.56	
	1	1	1X100 CP	EA	BV VIT E 1MIU SOFTGEL	123463	30761030520	OT	.00	10.32	10.32	NET
S	1	0	1X150 CHE	EA	CALCIUM ANTACID TB FRUIT 500MG	693200	30904641292	OT	3.40	1.55	.00	Short
	1	1	1X30 GM CRE	EA	FLUOCINONIDE CR .05% 30GM	168666	51672125302	RX	91.10	34.50	34.50	Contract
	3	3	1X50 CT STR	EA	HW TRUE TRACK TEST STRIPS 50CT	546754	02129200455	OT	28.51	19.00	57.00	NET
	2	2	1X30 TAB	EA	JANUVIA TABS 25MG	393348	00006022131	RX	436.08	345.23	690.46	Contract
	1	1	1X100 TBC	EA	LITHIUM CARB 450MG ER	287201	00054002025	RX	53.69	21.35	21.35	Contract
	1	1	1X500 TB1	EA	MUCINEX ER EXPECT TAB 600MG	254060	36382400850	OT	218.61	127.31	127.31	Contract
	4	4	1X30 CP2	EA	NAMENDA XR CAP 28MG	639880	00456342833	RX	424.80	345.15	1380.60	Contract

To the extent that this invoice or statement contains a discount, rebate, or credit, you may be obligated to report this discount, rebate, or credit along with other pertinent information to the Department of Health and Human Services or other government agencies under 42 C.F.R. Sec. 1001.952*h)(l).

RX	OTC:	DEA Sched:	Misc:	TOTAL:

A: Automatic Shipment   B: From Backorder   K: Mfr. can't supply   M: Discontinued by Mfr.   X: Discontinued by SDC   S: Short-please reorder   W: Will follow

LAB 45

Control Substance Report

▪ Introduction

Certain medications are designated as a ***narcotic***, ***controlled substance***, or ***scheduled drug*** and are placed in categories I through IV by the U.S. Food and Drug Administration (FDA). The following medications are some examples:

- CI—lysergic acid diethylamide (LSD), cocaine, heroin
- CII—Demerol, oxycodone, methadone, codeine, Vicodin
- CIII—Tylenol/codeine (#2, 3, 4)
- CIV—Valium, Ativan, phenobarbital
- CV—Robitussin AC, Phenergan with codeine *(This category of controlled medications requires a log entry at the time of dispensing.)*

Each group has special handling, inventory, and documentation requirements. Each pharmacy or dispensing facility must keep accurate records of all dispensed controlled drugs in these categories, and, as a pharmacy technician, you will be involved in this process under a pharmacist's supervision.

MEDICATION SAFETY CONSIDERATION

Always be aware of **BOTH** the state and federal law updates on dispensing activities and record-keeping requirements for controlled drugs. A drug may be considered a controlled substance in your state but may not be classified as such federally.

▪ Lab Objectives

In this Lab, you will:

- Discuss several common terms for controlled drugs and examples of medications within.
- Learn how to create a pharmacy business report that details the inventory and dispensing activity of controlled medications in the pharmacy.

▪ Scenario

Working in a community pharmacy, the managing pharmacist is reconciling the CII logbook. He needs to confirm that the exact count of a medication found in the narcotic cabinet matches what should be in the computer inventory. A discrepancy is found in Hydrocodone/APAP 7.5/3.25 mg. The CII logbook indicates that the pharmacy dispensed a total of 90 tablets since January. The pharmacist has asked for help in verifying the patients that were dispensed this medication and the amount to each. He will then reconcile the CII log to match the current inventory.

MEDICATION SAFETY CONSIDERATION

Most pharmacies keep controlled medications in a special place or cabinet for storage and perform a **PERPETUAL** inventory, which means every time a drug is removed, the exact inventory is corrected at that time.

▪ Pre Lab Information

Using your stock bottles and narcotics cabinet, count the exact number of Hydrocodone/ APAP 7.5/3.25 mg tablets in stock.

Documentation

Now, you will create a report to identify what was dispensed and to which patients with dates and prescription numbers. Once completed, show your work.

■ Student Directions

Estimated completion time: 15 minutes

1. Read through the steps in the Lab before performing the Lab exercise.
2. After reading through the Lab, perform the required steps to generate a control drug report.
3. Complete the exercise at the end of the Lab.

STEPS TO CREATE A CONTROL DRUG REPORT

1. Access the main screen of Visual SuperScript.

2. Click on **REPORTS** from the menu toolbar located at the top of the screen.

3. Select **DRUG REPORTS** from the drop-down menu. Then select **CONTROL DRUG REPORT** from the expanded menu.

4. The *Control Drug Report* dialog box appears. Enter a 2-month date range in the *Date From* and *To* fields.

5. The *Drug Class* field will designate if the report will generate a list of Class/Schedule II drugs only: C2 Only; Class/Schedule III through Class/Schedule V: C3-C5 drugs; or all the drugs in the report: All (C2-C5) drugs. Click on the appropriate choice.

   Select All (C2-C5).

6. The *Sort By* field will designate the order in which the report should be arranged. Indicate how the report should be arranged: Fill Date, Drug Name, or Customer. Click on the appropriate choice.

   Select Drug Name.

7. Choose the appropriate *Report Layout*.

   Select Detail.

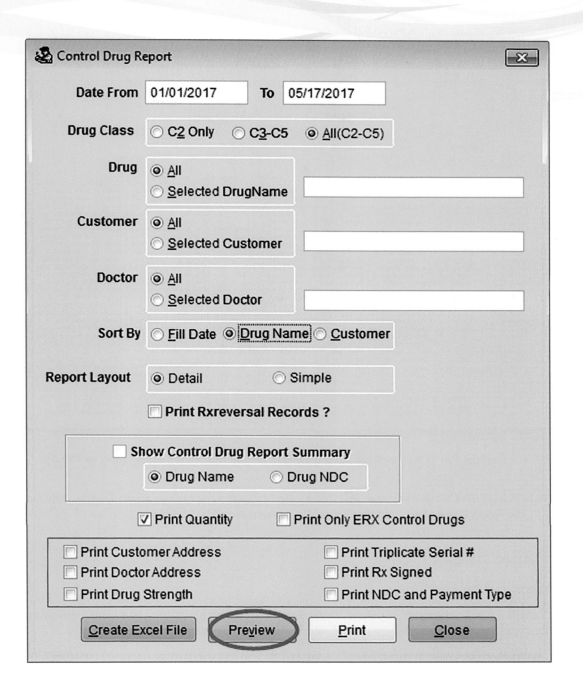

8. Click on **Preview** located at the bottom of the *Control Drug Report* dialog box. The selected *Control Drug Report* will open and appear on the screen, similar to the following example.

```
                          DAA EDUCATIONAL SOFTWARE              PAGE NO:1/2
                    369 HARVARD ST, SUITE 1,BROOKLINE, MA 02446
                              (617) 734-7366                     DATE:05/24/17


                         Controlled Drugs Report For Sched 2-5
                                (01/01/17 To 05/24/17)


Type Rx#   OrigDate FillDate Ref   Customer            Doctor            Drug                  Class Qty     RPh      DEA#      Sig
     183485 12/16/16 01/02/17 1/1  SLADE, KARINA       CHAPELLE, AKHI    ACETAMINOPHEN-COD #3   C3   56.00 RM/RMFC1234258 TAKE 1 TABLET BY MOUTH EVERY 6
     186332 01/04/17 01/04/17 0/0  CUNNINGTON, KEITH   MAHADEO, DEEPAK   ACETAMINOPHEN-COD #3   C3   90.00 RM/RMBB1234056 TAKE 1 TABLET BY MOUTH EVERY 4-6
     186369 01/04/17 01/04/17 0/2  MULLIGAN, GARY      BHAGWATI, MONIKA  ACETAMINOPHEN-COD #3   C3   45.00 RM/RMBB1234210 TAKE 1 TABLET BY MOUTH TWICE DAILY
     186525 04/04/17 04/04/17 0/1  JONES, SHIRLEY      NOBEL, ALFRED     ACETAMINOPHEN-COD #3   C3   60.00 IMR AN7321235 TAKE 2 TABLETS BY MOUTH EVERY 4-6
     186240 01/02/17 01/03/17 0/0  SANFORD, CORINE     CHIHARA, MATT     ALPRAZOLAM 0.25 MG     C4   30.00 RM/RMFC1234359 TAKE 1 TABLET BY MOUTH DAILY FOR
     186257 01/04/17 01/04/17 0/2  SOTOMAYOR, LUIS     DOSCH, RAMEZ      ALPRAZOLAM 1 MG TABLET C4   60.00 RM/RMAD1234929 TAKE 1 TABLET BY MOUTH TWICE DAILY
     186262 01/04/17 01/04/17 0/3  TOMEI, DENELLE      DOSCH, RAMEZ      ALPRAZOLAM 1 MG TABLET C4   30.00 RM/RMAD1234929 TAKE 1 TABLET BY MOUTH ONCE DAILY
     178432 11/14/16 01/02/17 0/3  DEBEERS, TERRENCE   ZABARSKI, MICHAEL ALPRAZOLAM 2 MG TABLET C4   60.00 RM/RMMA1234400 TAKE 1 TABLET BY MOUTH TWICE DAILY
     185878 01/02/17 01/02/17 0/1  WHITAKER, GLORIA    CRUSOE, JONATHAN  ALPRAZOLAM 2 MG TABLET C4   60.00 RM/RMFC1234068 TAKE 1 TABLET BY MOUTH EVERY 12
     185900 01/02/17 01/02/17 0/1  CARROLLTON,         CRUSOE, JONATHAN  ALPRAZOLAM 2 MG TABLET C4   60.00 RM/RMFC1234068 TAKE 1 TABLET BY MOUTH TWICE DAILY
     186336 12/25/16 01/04/17 0/0  WALKER, RONALD      SPERLING, MARY    ALPRAZOLAM 2 MG TABLET C4   60.00 RM/RMMS1234943 TAKE 1 TABLET BY MOUTH TWICE DAILY
     186395 01/04/17 01/04/17 0/0  VICKERS, CAMELIA    CRUSOE, JONATHAN  ALPRAZOLAM 2 MG TABLET C4   60.00 RM/RMFC1234068 TAKE 1 TABLET BY MOUTH TWICE DAILY
     186252 01/03/17 01/04/17 0/0  SMITH, RODNEY       PASCHAL, JOSEPH   BUPRENORPHIN-NALOXON 8-2 C3 30.00 RM/RMAD1234929 PLACE 1 TABLET UNDER THE TONGUE
     186428 01/04/17 01/04/17 0/2  BROWN, TORRES       DOSCH, RAMEZ      CLONAZEPAM 1 MG TABLET C4   30.00 RM/RMAD1234929 TAKE 1 TABLET BY MOUTH AT BEDTIME
     186461 03/14/17 03/14/17 0/3  WILLETT, TANYA      MARQUETTE, MAURA  CLONAZEPAM 1 MG TABLET C4   30.00 IMR MM1234905 TAKE 1 TABLET BY MOUTH ONCE DAILY
     186479 04/04/17 04/04/17 0/0  JACKSON, RONALD     ANDERSON, BARRY   HYDROCODONE-IBUPROFEN  C2   60.00 IMR AA1126374 TAKE 1 TABLET BY MOUTH TWICE DAILY
     186225 01/03/17 01/03/17 0/0  ANDERSON, GENE      TILLMAN, PETER    HYDROCODONE/APAP 5/325 C2   40.00 RM/RMFT1234878 TAKE 1 TABLET BY MOUTH TWICE DAILY
     185899 01/02/17 01/02/17 0/0  CARROLLTON,         CRUSOE, JONATHAN  HYDROCODONE/APAP 7.5/325 C2 60.00 RM/RMFC1234068 TAKE 1 TABLET BY MOUTH EVERY 12
     186056 12/29/16 01/03/17 0/0  PARKHURST, BARBARA  MCCLAIN, MICHELLE HYDROCODONE/APAP 7.5/325 C2 30.00 RM/RMMM1234222 TAKE 1 TABLET BY MOUTH TWICE DAILY
     186459 03/21/17 03/21/17 0/5  BURTON, LASHAWNA    HALEY, MARIA      KLONOPIN 1 MG TABLET   C4   30.00 IMR MH1234145 TAKE 1 TABLET BY MOUTH ONCE DAILY
     184445 12/22/16 01/02/17 0/0  ADAMS, MARGARET     DOSCH, RAMEZ      LORAZEPAM 1 MG TABLET  C4   30.00 RM/RMAD1234929 TAKE 1 TABLET BY MOUTH AT BEDTIME
     179334 11/18/16 01/03/17 1/2  SMITH, RODNEY       JABRI, AYMAN      LORAZEPAM 2 MG TABLET  C4   60.00 RM/RMBJ1234397 TAKE 1 TABLET BY MOUTH TWICE DAILY
     177402 11/07/16 01/07/16 1/1  VICKERS, CAMELIA    CRUSOE, JONATHAN  LYRICA 50 MG CAPSULE   C5   90.00 RM/RMFC1234068 TAKE 1 CAPSULE BY MOUTH 3 TIMES A
     171370 10/01/16 01/02/17 3/2  BEASON, PATRINA     LAKHANI, DEEPAK   PHENOBARBITAL 32.4 MG  C4   60.00 RM/RMEL1234931 TAKE 1 TABLET BY MOUTH TWICE DAILY
     186359 01/04/17 01/04/17 0/0  PULLMAN, RICHARD    TILLMAN, PETER    SUBOXONE 8MG/2MG SL FILM C3  4.00 RM/RMFT1234878 TAKE 1 FILM UNDER THE TONGUE EVERY
     186363 01/04/17 01/04/17 0/0  CARTIER, DAVID      TILLMAN, PETER    SUBOXONE 8MG/2MG SL FILM C3 30.00 RM/RMFT1234878 TAKE 1 FILM UNDER THE TONGUE DAILY
     186399 01/04/17 01/04/17 0/0  TAYLOR, WILLIAM     TILLMAN, PETER    SUBOXONE 8MG/2MG SL FILM C3 14.00 RM/RMFT1234878 TAKE 1 FILM UNDER THE TONGUE TWICE
     177403 01/02/17 01/02/17 1/1  VICKERS, CAMELIA    CRUSOE, JONATHAN  TRAMADOL HCL 50 MG     C4   90.00 RM/RMFC1234068 TAKE 1 TABLET BY MOUTH EVERY 8
     186245 01/03/17 01/03/17 0/3  VENZIANO, JUANITA   CRUSOE, JONATHAN  TRAMADOL HCL 50 MG     C4   60.00 RM/RMFC1234068 TAKE 1 TABLET BY MOUTH EVERY 12
     174374 10/18/16 01/04/17 2/3  LITTLEFIELD,        AZMI, HUMA        TRAMADOL HCL 50 MG     C4   60.00 RM/RMBA1234537 TAKE 1 TABLET BY MOUTH 3 TIMES A
```

9. Click on the **Print Report** 🖨 icon located at the top right of the *Report Designer* toolbar.

10. Click on the **Close Preview** icon located at the top right of the *Report Designer* toolbar. The report is closed out, and the *Control Drug Report* dialog box returns.

EXERCISE

Task

Compile a detailed listing of dispensed Alprazolam 2 mg from 01/01/2017 to 03/01/2017, following the steps in this Lab. Print the report, and submit it for verification.

1. What is the number of Alprazolam 2 mg tablets that were dispensed from the pharmacy on 01/02/2017?

2. What are the three *Control Drug Report* sort choices?

QUICK CHALLENGE

You are becoming more familiar with the Visual SuperScript software system. Can you find the main menu option that will print a list of top-selling drugs?

1. Print a *Top-Selling Drug Report* listing the 10 top-selling drugs by average wholesale price (AWP) from 01/01/2017 through 06/30/2017. Submit the report to your instructor for verification.

2. What is the name of the top-selling or top-performing drugs for this period?

3. Name one example from each classification of controlled drugs.

LAB 46

Daily Prescription Log Report

■ Introduction

You have completed a report for all controlled substances filled during a specified period, and now in this Lab, we will run the report to show all of the prescriptions processed during this time. For a community setting, a daily report of all of the medications filled, by customer, is usually automatically generated after hours. Depending on each state law, the report can be paper or kept electronically.

■ Lab Objectives

In this Lab, you will:

- Demonstrate how to create a report that summarizes the pharmacy dispensing records.
- Continue to use the database for inventory and record-keeping purposes.

■ Scenario

It is the end of a busy day at your pharmacy, and the pharmacist has asked you to run the daily log report.

■ Pre Lab Information

As part of the daily tasks in a pharmacy, a report with the day's prescription activity is maintained. Although this is often automatically set as a "back-up" computer report printed after hours, you will print a physical report in this scenario.

■ Student Directions

Estimated completion time: 20 minutes

1. Read through the steps in the Lab before performing the Lab exercise.
2. After reading through the Lab, perform the required steps to generate a daily prescription log report.
3. Complete the exercise at the end of the Lab.

STEPS TO CREATE A DAILY PRESCRIPTION LOG REPORT

1. Access the main screen of Visual SuperScript.

2. Click on **REPORTS** from the menu toolbar located at the top of the screen.

3. Select **DAILY LOG REPORTS** from the drop-down menu. Then select **DAILY RX LOG** from the expanded menu.

Documentation

4. The *Daily Rx Log* dialog box appears and defaults to the **MAIN OPTIONS** tab. The *Select* section of the dialog box offers three choices on information that will be included in the daily prescription log report: All Prescriptions, New Prescriptions Only, or Refills Only. Click on the appropriate choice.

Select All Prescriptions.

5. Enter a 1-month date range in *Include Records From* and *To* fields.

6. The *Aggregation Type* field allows for formatting choices in the report. Click on the appropriate choice.

Choose Separate Each Day.

 LAB TIP

Choose Separate Each Day if the report should have prescription information from each date on a separate page. Choose Combined for Period if the report should have prescription information flow from one page to another, regardless of the date.

7. Click on the *Show Cost Using* check box. Designate if the report should be generated to show the average wholesale price (AWP) for prescriptions dispensed during the selected date(s) or the Acquisition cost of the medications dispensed. Click on the appropriate choice.

Select AWP.

8. The *Sort By* data entry field allows four different formats in sorting or arranging the Daily Prescription log report: Fill Date, Drug Class, Rx #, PCN No, or Pay Type. Click on the appropriate choice.

Choose FILL DATE.

9. Click on the **ADVANCE OPTIONS** tab. Choose the amount of information that should be included on the daily prescription log report in the *Detail Level* section. Click on the appropriate choice.

Choose Detail Level Three.

 HINT

Detail Level One is the basic report that provides prescription information. Detail Level Two provides the patient's address in addition to the basic information. Detail Level Three provides the patient and prescriber's addresses, as well as the National Drug Code (NDC) number of the dispensed medication in addition to the basic information.

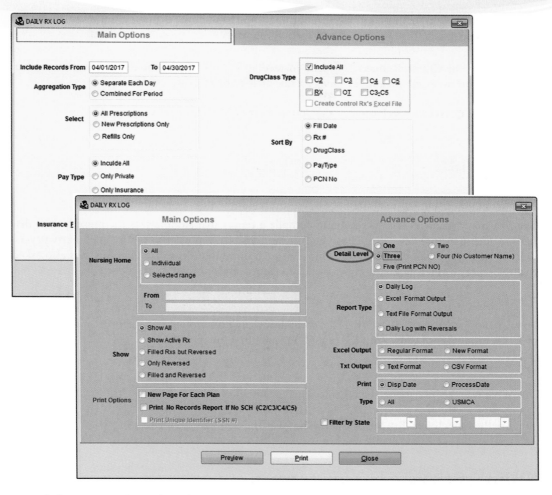

10. Click **Preview** located on the bottom of the *Daily Rx Log* dialog box. The selected Daily Prescription Log Report will open and appear on the screen.

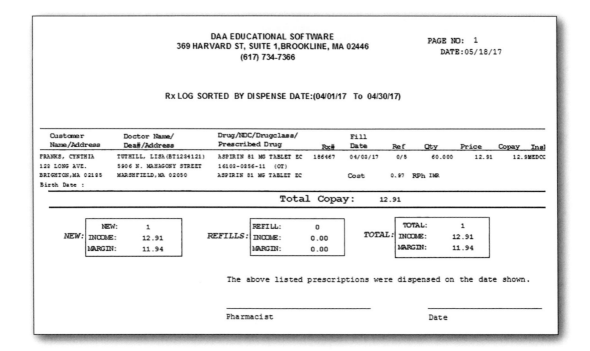

Documentation

11. Click on the **PRINT REPORT** icon located at the top right of the *Report Designer* toolbar. Be sure to print only the pages necessary for this report.

12. Click on the **CLOSE REPORT** ⬚ icon located at the top right of the *Report Designer* toolbar. The report is closed out and the *Daily Rx Log* dialog box returns.

13. Click on **CLOSE** button located at the bottom of the *Daily Rx Log* dialog box.

EXERCISE

■ Scenario

The pharmacy manager has asked you to compile a report that summarizes the prescriptions dispensed during the previous year. The manager would like the report arranged by third-party payers. The report should include the NDC number of each dispensed drug. The manager has also asked that the report be filed as a hard-copy or backup record in case of a system failure.

Task

Following the steps presented in this Lab, compile a Daily Prescription Log Report that will meet the pharmacy manager's needs. Print the report, and submit it for verification.

1. Who are the third-party payers?

2. What was the fill date for the One-Touch Test Strips?

3. Are the One-Touch Test Strips listed as an over-the-counter (OTC) item or a prescription?

QUICK CHALLENGE

1. You are now familiar with the steps of generating a business report. Can you compile a *Top Selling Drugs Report* for the previous 6 months? Submit the printed report for verification.

> ◎ **HINT**
>
> Select an item by left-clicking on the item with your mouse.

Documentation

LAB 47

Customer History Report

■ Introduction

In addition to a complete report for **ALL** customer prescriptions filled at a pharmacy, an additional task for the pharmacy technician includes a request from a customer or an outside provider for an individual prescription history. Because of customer privacy (the Health Insurance Portability and Accountability Act [HIPAA]), a report containing information about other patients cannot be shared with a single patient; consequently, an individual report that spans a specified period is appropriate. This type of report could be needed for reimbursement from a health reimbursement account (HRA) or for a medical provider wanting to perform a complete review of a patient's medications. For example, the patient is told to bring a complete list of medications to a specialist appointment, and you are asked to print the most recent profile for him or her.

MEDICATION SAFETY CONSIDERATION

Maintaining the most accurate record of the patient's medications, including vitamins and over-the-counter (OTC) medications, as well as other pertinent information in their profile (e.g., allergies, disease states), is extremely important. Often dose adjustment or other similar decisions and audit information are made on the basis of this drug review.

■ Lab Objectives

In this Lab, you will:

- Discuss the reasons why a patient's specific history of prescriptions filled would be needed rather than a daily log.
- Demonstrate how to create a pharmacy business report that details the patient or customer prescription history.

■ Scenario

Dr. Adams' office has called and is requesting a faxed copy of all the medications for Floyd Ellis (date of birth [DOB]: 12/4/23) that have been filled within the last 2 months. He is at the physician's office for a preoperative visit and forgot to bring his list to the appointment.

■ Pre Lab Information

To ensure that the information is correct, verify the DOB in your profile and then follow the steps on the next page to run the report.

■ Student Directions

Estimated completion time: 15 minutes

1. Read through the steps in the Lab before performing the Lab exercise.
2. After reading through the Lab, perform the required steps to generate a customer history report.
3. Complete the exercise at the end of the Lab.

1. Access the main screen of Visual SuperScript.

2. Click on **REPORTS** from the menu toolbar located at the top of the screen.

3. Select **CUSTOMER REPORTS** from the drop-down menu. Then select **CUSTOMER HISTORY** from the expanded menu.

4. The *Customer History* dialog box appears. Notice that the insertion point is in the first data entry field, *Date From*. Type in the date that the Customer History Report should start.

Key in *01/20/2017*.

5. Type in the date that the Customer History Report should end in the *To* data entry field.

Key in *12/31/2017*.

6. The *Show* field will designate if the report should be generated to show the Copay amount for the medications or the actual Price of the medications. Click on the appropriate choice.

Select Copay.

7. The *Format* field will designate whether the report should be generated in an Insurance format or an NHome (nursing home) format. Select Insurance format unless the patient is a resident of a nursing home. Click on the appropriate choice.

Select Insurance.

8. Select the *New Page for Each Customer* field if individual pages are desired.

9. The *For* data field offers several different choices in generating the Customer History Report. Select one of the five choices in which the Customer History Report will be generated. Click on the appropriate choice.

Select Individual Customer.

10. The *Name* data entry field will ask for the customer's name or the name of the insurance plan. The required information depends on the selection made in Step 9. Type in the appropriate information.

Key in *ELL* for Ellis, Floyd.

 HINT

Type the first three letters of the customer's last name, and hit **ENTER**. The *Customer Lookup* dialog box will appear, and you can choose the customer from this box.

11. Choose the print layout for the report.

Select Portrait.

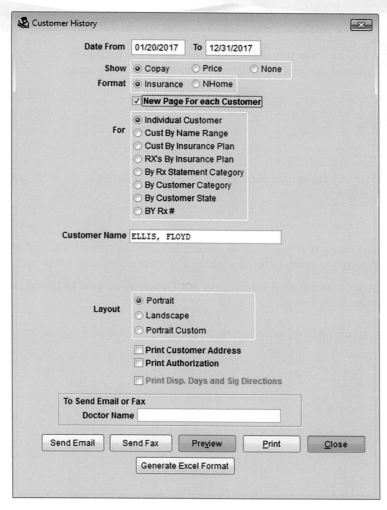

12. Click on **Preview** located the bottom of the *Customer History* dialog box. The selected Customer History Report will open and appear on the screen.

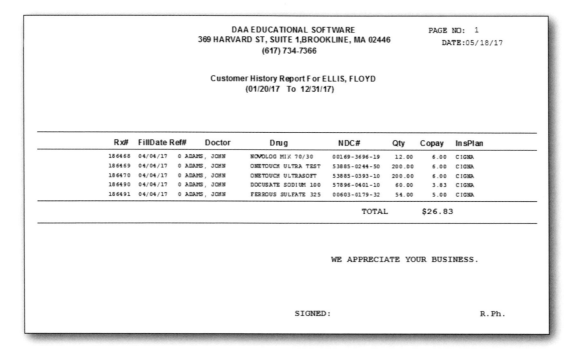

13. Click on the **PRINT REPORT** 🖨 icon located at the top right of the *Report Designer* toolbar.

14. Click on the **CLOSE PREVIEW** 📲 icon located at the top right of the *Report Designer* toolbar. The report is closed out, and the *Customer History* dialog box returns.

EXERCISE

▪ Scenario

Mr. Brian Davidson calls your pharmacy asking for a detailed listing of the medications that he has purchased so far this year.

Task

Compile a detailed listing of Mr. Davidson's medications for the current year to date, following the steps from the *Reporting Customer History* exercise. Print the report, and submit it for verification.

1. What is the total out-of-pocket expense that Mr. Davidson has paid to your pharmacy this year for prescription medications?

2. How many capsules did Mr. Davidson receive on his prescription for clavaris?

LAB 48

United States Drug Enforcement Administration Form

▪ Introduction

The United States Drug Enforcement Administration (DEA) enforces the controlled substance laws and regulations of the United States. There are five ratings of controlled substances: C-I, C-II, C-III, C-IV, and C-V. The ratings refer to the potential for abuse, with C-I being the highest. C-I drugs have no accepted medical purpose and a very high potential for abuse; consequently, these drugs cannot be prescribed. The following table provides the details for each level of a controlled substance. DEA Form 222 must be completed to order or transfer C-II drugs from a distributor.

Type of Medication

DRUG LEVEL	GENERIC NAME	TRADE NAME	POTENTIAL FOR ABUSE
C-I		LSD Cocaine (crack or street) Mescaline Heroine	Have no accepted medical use in the United States. Potential for abuse is very high.
C-II	amphetamines codeine fentanyl hydrocodone/APAP hydrocodone/ibuprofen hydromorphone meperidine methadone methylphenidate morphine opium oxycodone/APAP oxycodone/ASA	Demerol Dilaudid Duragesic Percocet Percodan Ritalin Vicodin Vicoprofen	Potential for abuse is high. Are used for medicinal purposes. Abuse may lead to severe psychologic or physical dependence.
C-III	acetaminophen/codeine #2, #3, #4	Tylenol	Potential for abuse under this schedule is less than that of controlled substances under C-II. Abuse may lead to moderate or low physical dependence or high psychologic dependence. Most schedule III drugs are combination narcotics.
C-IV	chlordiazepoxide diazepam flurazepam lorazepam pentazocine phenobarbital	Ativan Dalmane Librium Talwin Valium	Potential for abuse is low, compared with C-III drugs. Abuse may lead to limited physical or psychologic dependence.
C-V	diphenoxylate/atropine guaifenesin/codeine promethazine/codeine	Diocalm Lomotil Phenergan Robitussin AC	Low potential for abuse compared with C-IV drugs; abuse may lead to limited physical or psychological dependence.

APAP, Acetyl-p-aminophenol (acetaminophen); *ASA*, acetylsalicylic acid (aspirin); *LSD*, lysergic acid diethylamide.
From *Mosby's pharmacy technician: principles and practice*, ed 4, St Louis, 2016, Mosby.

Documentation

Select a C-II drug from the table, and complete DEA Form 222 as though your pharmacy is ordering that particular drug. A printable copy of the form is available on the Evolve Resources site.

Sample DEA Form 222							
See Reverse of PURCHASER'S Copy for Instructions	No order form may be issued for Schedule I and II substances unless completed application form has been received (21 CRF 1305.04)					OMB APPROVAL NO. 1117-0010	
TO:	STREET ADDRESS						
CITY AND STATE		DATE		TO BE FILLED IN BY SUPPLIER			
				SUPPLIER DEA REGISTRATION NO.			
	TO BE FILLED IN BY PURCHASER						
	No. of Packages	Size of Package	Name of Item	National Drug Code		Packaging Shipped	Date Shipped
1							
2							
3							
4							
5							
6							
7							
8							
9							
10							
◀ LAST LINE COMPLETED	(MUST BE 10 OR LESS)		SIGNATURE OF PURCHASER OR ATTORNEY OR AGENT				
Date Issued		DEA Registration No.		Name and Address of Registrant			
Schedules							
Registered as a		No. of this Order Form					
DEA Form 222 (Oct. 1992)	US OFFICIAL ORDER FORMS - SCHEDULES I & II DRUG ENFORCEMENT ADMINISTRATION SUPPLIER'S Copy 1						

Courtesy Drug Enforcement Administration, Washington, DC.

Documentation

LAB 49

Medication Therapy Management Report

■ Introduction

Patients often take a variety of drugs (e.g., prescription, over-the-counter medications, supplements). Medication records, such as the example included in this Lab, help patients keep track of all of their drugs, enabling them to provide the correct information to their physicians.

EXERCISE

Complete the form in this Lab. A printable copy of the form is available on the Evolve Resources site.

<table>
<tr><td colspan="7" align="center">MY MEDICATION RECORD</td></tr>
<tr><td colspan="4">Name: _____</td><td colspan="3">Birth date: _____</td></tr>
<tr><td colspan="7">Phone number: _____</td></tr>
<tr><td colspan="4">Emergency Contact</td><td colspan="3">Pharmacy</td></tr>
<tr><td colspan="4">Name: _____
Relationship: _____
Phone Number: _____</td><td colspan="3">Name:_____
Phone Number:_____</td></tr>
<tr><td colspan="4" rowspan="2">Primary Care Physician

Name: _____
Phone Number: _____</td><td colspan="3">Allergies (list below)</td></tr>
<tr><td colspan="3"></td></tr>
<tr><td colspan="4">Other Physicians</td><td colspan="3">Medical Conditions (list below)</td></tr>
<tr><td colspan="4">Name: _____
Specialty: _____
Phone Number: _____
Name: _____
Specialty: _____
Phone Number: _____</td><td colspan="3"></td></tr>
<tr><td>Drug Name</td><td>Dose</td><td>Taking for...</td><td>When do I take it?</td><td>How much do I take?</td><td>Start and End Dates</td><td>Special information or Instructions</td></tr>
<tr><td>Tylenol</td><td>500 mg</td><td>Pain</td><td>Twice a day: once in the morning and once in the evening</td><td>1 tablet</td><td>11/5/16-ongoing</td><td>Take with food</td></tr>
<tr><td></td><td></td><td></td><td></td><td></td><td></td><td></td></tr>
<tr><td></td><td></td><td></td><td></td><td></td><td></td><td></td></tr>
<tr><td></td><td></td><td></td><td></td><td></td><td></td><td></td></tr>
<tr><td></td><td></td><td></td><td></td><td></td><td></td><td></td></tr>
<tr><td colspan="7">Include all of your medications, including prescription drugs, over-the-counter drugs, herbal supplements, and vitamins.</td></tr>
</table>

LAB 50

Medication Reconciliation Forms

■ Introduction

Medication reconciliation is important in preventing medication errors. Inpatient and outpatient medication reconciliation forms are two of the tools used in medication reconciliation. Examples of these forms are included in this Lab, and printable versions can be found on the Evolve Resources site. Steps on how to add and edit information in a patient's profile can be found in Lab 32.

INPATIENT

From *Workbook and lab manual for Mosby's pharmacy technician: principles and practice*, ed 4, St Louis, 2016, Mosby.

Documentation

MEDICATION RECONCILIATION FORM

Patient Name: _____ Doctor: _____

DOB: _____ Age/Gender: _____ Admit Date: _____

Daily Scheduled Medications

Drug Name and Dosage	Frequency	Last Taken	No Longer Taking	Comments
1.				
2.				
3.				
4.				
5.				
6.				
7.				
8.				
9.				
10.				

OTC Medication and Herbal Supplements

1.				
2.				
3.				
4.				
5.				
6.				
7.				
8.				
9.				
10.				

NOTES

NOTES

NOTES

NOTES